Aquaculture Biosecurity

Prevention, Control, and Eradication of Aquatic Animal Disease

AF775386

Aquaculture Biosecurity

Prevention, Control, and Eradication of Aquatic Animal Disease

Edited by

A. David Scarfe

Assistant Director, Scientific Activities
American Veterinary Medical Association
Schaumburg, Illinois, USA

Cheng-Sheng Lee

Director, Aquaculture Interchange Program
Oceanic Institute, Waimanalo, Hawaii, USA

Patricia J. O'Bryen

Project Manager, Aquaculture Interchange Program
Oceanic Institute, Waimanalo, Hawaii, USA

WORLD AQUACULTURE SOCIETY

NOAA
NATIONAL OCEANIC AND ATMOSPHERIC ADMINISTRATION
U.S. DEPARTMENT OF COMMERCE

Blackwell Publishing

Oceanic Institute
An Affiliate of Hawai'i Pacific University

©2006 Blackwell Publishing
All rights reserved

Blackwell Publishing Professional
2121 State Avenue, Ames, Iowa 50014, USA
Orders: 1-800-862-6657
Office: 1-515-292-0140
Fax: 1-515-292-3348
Web site: www.blackwellprofessional.com

Blackwell Publishing Ltd
9600 Garsington Road, Oxford OX4 2DQ, UK
Tel.: +44 (0)1865 776868

Blackwell Publishing Asia
550 Swanston Street, Carlton, Victoria 3053, Australia
Tel.: +61 (0)3 8359 1011

Authorization to photocopy items for internal or personal use, or the internal or personal use of specific clients, is granted by Blackwell Publishing, provided that the base fee is paid directly to the Copyright Clearance Center, 222 Rosewood Drive, Danvers, MA 01923. For those organizations that have been granted a photocopy license by CCC, a separate system of payments has been arranged. The fee codes for users of the Transactional Reporting Service are ISBN-13: 978-0-8138-0539-9/2006.

First edition, 2006

Library of Congress Cataloging-in-Publication Data

Aquaculture biosecurity : prevention, control, and eradication of aquatic animal disease / edited by A. David Scarfe, Cheng-Sheng Lee, Patricia J. O'Bryen. – 1st ed.
p. cm.
Includes index.
ISBN-13: 978-0-8138-0539-9 (alk. paper)
ISBN-10: 0-8138-0539-2 (alk. paper)
1. Fishes—Diseases—Prevention. 2. Shellfish—Diseases—Prevention.
I. Scarfe, A. David. II. Lee, Cheng-Sheng. III. O'Bryen, P. J. (Patricia J.)
SH171.A67 2006
639.8—dc22

2005016403

The last digit is the print number: 9 8 7 6 5 4 3 2

Contents

Contributors vii

Preface xi

1 Aquaculture Biosecurity: The View and Approaches of the OIE (World Organisation for Animal Health) Regarding Prevention and Control of Aquatic Animal Diseases 3
Eva-Maria Bernoth

2 Biosecurity in Aquaculture: International Agreements and Instruments, their Compliance, Prospects, and Challenges for Developing Countries 9
Rohana P. Subasinghe and Melba G. Bondad-Reantaso

3 Regional Approach to Aquatic Animal Health Management—Views and Programs of the Network of Aquaculture Centres in Asia–Pacific 17
C.V. Mohan and Melba G. Bondad-Reantaso

4 Canada's Approach to Aquatic Animal Biosecurity: Experience and Evolution 31
Sharon E. McGladdery and Richard E. Zurbrigg

5 The U.S. Fish & Wildlife Service's "Aquatic Animal Health Policy": Innovative Approaches to Managing Diseases in Traditional and Special-Case Aquatic Animals 55
Thomas A. Bell, J. Scott Foott, Kathy Clemens, Susan Gutenberger, Ray Brunson, John Thoesen, Rick Nelson, Norm Heil, John Coll, and Crystal Hudson

6 Wisconsin's Veterinary Approach to Fish Health 69
Myron J. Kebus

7 Harmonized, Standardized, and Flexible National Frameworks for Ensuring Diagnostic Data and Test Result Validity: A Critical Need for Aquatic Animal Health Diagnostic Systems and for Biosecurity in Aquaculture 77
Ann L. Wiegers, Jerry R. Heidel, and A. David Scarfe

8 Disinfectants, Disinfection, and Biosecurity in Aquaculture 91
G. Russell Danner and Peter Merrill

9 Aquatic Animal Health Surveillance 129
F. Chris Baldock, Angus R. Cameron, and Nigel R. Perkins

10 Biosecurity at the Farm Level—How to Create a State of Mind 149
Paul Hardy-Smith

11 Elements of an Aquatic Animal Health Program—Infectious Hematopoietic Necrosis in Farmed Atlantic Salmon in British Columbia 155
Grace A. Karreman

12 A Preliminary Investigation of the Relationship between Infected Cage Removal Speed and Resultant Spread of Infectious Salmon Anemia on Atlantic Salmon Farms in Maine, U.S.A., and New Brunswick, Canada 165
Lori Gustafson, Stephen Ellis, Leighanne Hawkins, Mark Moore, Teresa Robinson, and Dan MacPhee

Index 173

Contributors

F. Chris Baldock AusVet Animal Health Services, 19 Brereton Street, P.O. Box 3180, South Brisbane, Queensland, 4101, Australia.

Thomas A. Bell U.S. Fish & Wildlife Service, Division of the National Fish Hatchery System, Aquatic Animal Drug Approval Partnership Program, 4050 Bridger Canyon Road, Bozeman, Montana 59715, USA.

Eva-Maria Bernoth Australian Government Department of Agriculture, Fisheries and Forestry, Office of the Chief Veterinary Officer, GPO Box 858, Canberra, ACT 2601, Australia.

Melba G. Bondad-Reantaso Food and Agriculture Organization of the United Nations, Fisheries Department, Viale delle Terme di Caracalla, 00100 Rome, Italy.

Ray Brunson U.S. Fish & Wildlife Service, Olympia Fish Health Center, 3704 Griffin Lane S.E., Suite 101, Olympia, Washington 98501, USA.

Angus R. Cameron AusVet Animal Health Services, 19 Brereton Street, P.O. Box 3180, South Brisbane, Queensland, 4101, Australia.

Kathy Clemens U.S. Fish & Wildlife Service, Idaho Fish Health Center, P.O. Box 272, Orofino, Idaho 83544, USA.

John Coll U.S. Fish & Wildlife Service, Lamar Fish Health Center, P.O. Box 155, Lamar, Pennsylvania 16848, USA.

G. Russell Danner Fish Health Laboratory, Maine Department of Inland Fisheries and Wildlife, Rural Route 5, Box 81, Hatchery Road, Augusta, Maine 03440, USA.

Stephen Ellis USDA-APHIS Veterinary Services, 16 Deep Cove Road, Eastport, Maine 04631, USA.

J. Scott Foott U.S. Fish & Wildlife Service, California-Nevada Fish Health Center, 24411 Coleman Hatchery Road, Anderson, California 96007, USA.

Lori Gustafson USDA-APHIS Veterinary Services, 16 Deep Cove Road, Eastport, Maine 04631, USA.

Susan Gutenberger U.S. Fish & Wildlife Service, Lower Columbia Fish Health Center, 61552 State Route 14, Underwood, Washington 98651, USA.

Paul Hardy-Smith Panaquatic Health Solutions, 26A Liddiard Street, Hawthorn, Victoria, 3122, Australia.

Leighanne Hawkins Maritime Veterinary Services 12-2 clinch St., St. George, NB, E5C 3C8, Canada.

Jerry R. Heidel Oregon State University, Magruder Hall 134, Corvallis, Oregon 97331, USA.

Norm Heil U.S. Fish & Wildlife Service, Warm Springs Fish Health Center, 5308 Spring Street, Warm Springs, Georgia 31830, USA.

Crystal Hudson U.S. Fish & Wildlife Service, Bozeman Fish Health Center, 920 Technology Boulevard, Suite G, Bozeman, Montana 59718, USA.

Grace A. Karreman Pacific Marine Veterinary Services, 3000 Andre Road, Nanaimo, British Columbia, Canada V9R 6X2.

Myron J. Kebus Wisconsin Department of Agriculture, Trade and Consumer Protection, Division of Animal Health, 2811 Agriculture Drive, Madison, Wisconsin 53708-8911, USA.

Dan MacPhee Maritime Veterinary Services, St. George, New Brunswick, Canada.

Sharon E. McGladdery Fisheries and Oceans Canada, Science Branch, 200 Kent Street, Ottawa, Ontario, Canada K1A 0E6.

Peter Merrill Micro Technologies, Inc., 41 Main Street, Richmond, Maine 04357, USA.

C. V. Mohan Network of Aquaculture Centres in Asia–Pacific, Suraswadi Building, Department of Fisheries, Kasetsart University Campus, Ladyao, Jatujak, Bangkok 10900, Thailand.

Mark Moore Maritime Veterinary Services, St. George, New Brunswick, Canada.

Rick Nelson U.S. Fish & Wildlife Service, LaCrosse Fish Health Center, 555 Lester Avenue, Onalaska, Wisconsin 54650, USA.

Nigel R. Perkins AusVet Animal Health Services, 19 Brereton Street, P.O. Box 3180, South Brisbane, Queensland, 4101, Australia.

Teresa Robinson USDA-APHIS Veterinary Services, 16 Deep Cove Road, Eastport, Maine 04631, USA.

A. David Scarfe American Veterinary Medical Association, 1931 North Meacham Road, Suite 100, Schaumburg, Illinois 60173-4360, USA.

Rohana P. Subasinghe Fishery Resources Division, Fisheries Department, Food and Agriculture Organization of the United Nations, Viale delle Terme di Caracalla, 00100 Rome, Italy.

John Thoesen U.S. Fish & Wildlife Service, Pinetop Fish Health Center, P.O. Box 160, 1684 East White Mountain Boulevard, Suite 7, Pinetop, Arizona 85935, USA.

Ann L. Wiegers United States Department of Agriculture, Animal and Plant Health Inspection Service, Veterinary Services, Center for Veterinary Biologics-Policy, Evaluation, and Licensing, 510 S. 17th Street, Suite 104, Ames, Iowa 50010, USA.

Richard H. Zurbrigg Fisheries and Oceans Canada, Science Branch, 200 Kent Street, Ottawa, Ontario, Canada K1A 0E6.

Preface

Aquaculture loses millions of dollars in revenue annually to aquatic animal diseases. In response, stakeholders in aquaculture, from the individual farmer to policy-makers, are promoting and implementing biosecurity programs to combat the diseases responsible for these losses. Oceanic Institute (OI) and the American Veterinary Medical Association (AVMA) brought these diverse stakeholders together for a 3-day special session, "Aquaculture Biosecurity 2004," at the World Aquaculture Society (WAS) annual conference in Honolulu, Hawaii, March 1–5, 2004. The goal of the special session was to update information on the various approaches being taken and to identify what next steps are needed for implementing effective biosecurity programs from the farm level up. This book contains 12 of the 30 presentations given by the diverse stakeholders in their areas of expertise. This activity was conducted under a grant from the National Oceanic and Atmospheric Administration (NOAA) Office of Oceanic and Atmospheric Research (Grant #NA17RG2076) to OI and was supported by the AVMA and WAS.

To be effective, aquaculture biosecurity needs to establish an integrated approach between the farms and governments to exclude and combat aquatic animal diseases. Approaches being integrated and implemented at the international (World Organisation for Animal Health [OIE] and the Food and Agriculture Organization of the United Nations [FAO]) and the regional level (Network of Aquaculture Centres in Asia–Pacific [NACA]) are covered in Chapters 1–3. The OIE, with a membership of 166 countries in March 2004, publishes the *Aquatic Animal Health Code* and *Manual of Diagnostic Tests for Aquatic Animals* and updates them annually. The FAO has developed Codes of Conduct and best management practices throughout the world that result in increased profitability. The NACA works in conjunction with the OIE and the FAO to formulate biosecurity policy, with programs that focus on reducing the risk of disease transmission.

Canada's national Aquatic Animal Health Program (Chapter 4) was developed through partnerships at the national, regional, and producer levels, working together to address the health of both wild and aquaculture species. Their biosecurity issues include new species diversification and domestication and the potential for newly emerging diseases, the increased number of facilities and live transfers, a growth in consumer demand for healthy products, and more challenges from environmental groups.

In the United States, many government agencies are involved in aquaculture in different ways. The U.S. Department of Agriculture regulates all animal health, including aquatic animals. The NOAA Fisheries promotes good stewardship of national fisheries resources, and is calling for a dramatic increase in aquaculture in the next 20 years that may involve animal health. The U.S. Fish & Wildlife Service is responsible for threatened and endangered freshwater species, and has developed diagnostic procedures, husbandry practices, and risk assessment worksheets that are useful for biosecurity programs (Chapter 5). There is a need for harmonization among these government agencies and for biosecurity programs for the ornamental industry.

Most protection from disease in the United States is done at the state level, but import regulations also need to be harmonized. Many states have no regulations, some address only salmonids, and most regulations are inaccessible to producers. Wisconsin is one of the few states that address biosecurity and health programs for large numbers of freshwater species (Chapter 6), such as yellow perch, to issue health certificates for non-salmonid operations. Another area in need of harmonization for effective aquaculture biosecurity in the United States is in diagnostic data collecting and reporting and validity of test results (Chapter 7).

At the farm level, common themes are education, communication, and economics. This book provides information on the proper use of disinfectants (Chapter 8), aquatic animal health surveillance (Chapter 9), and how to raise farmer awareness and keep them informed about biosecurity issues (Chapter 10).

Case studies of two diseases affecting the salmon industry, infectious hematopoietic necrosis (IHN) and infectious salmon anemia (ISA), are described in Chapters 11 and 12, respectively. Industry response led to effective disease management in the IHN study. The ISA study points out the need for increased surveillance.

Aquaculture Biosecurity 2004 was the follow-up to a workshop on biosecurity held by OI in Honolulu in July 2001, and provided additional information for effective biosecurity programs against aquatic animal diseases. The session brought out the need for increased integration of biosecurity measures from the farm to the international level, identified some of the major issues that need to be addressed, and made recommendations on the next steps to be taken to ensure the profitability and sustainability of aquaculture.

We would like to express our thanks and appreciation to Dr. A. David Scarfe for his assistance in planning the special session and identifying presenters for Aquaculture Biosecurity 2004, to the contributing authors, to manuscript reviewers for their helpful comments and suggestions, and to Ms. Alcian Clegg for her valued assistance in preparing the manuscripts for review and publication.

Cheng-Sheng Lee and Patricia J. O'Bryen
Oceanic Institute, 41-202 Kalanianaole Hwy.
Waimanalo, Hawaii 96795, USA

Aquaculture Biosecurity

Prevention, Control, and Eradication of Aquatic Animal Disease

Chapter 1

Aquaculture Biosecurity: The View and Approaches of the OIE (World Organisation for Animal Health) Regarding Prevention and Control of Aquatic Animal Diseases

Eva-Maria Bernoth

Abstract

The OIE (World Organisation for Animal Health) is an intergovernmental organization, created in 1924. In March 2004, the OIE totaled 166 Member Countries. One of the main objectives of the OIE, within its mandate under the World Trade Organization Agreement on the Application of Sanitary and Phytosanitary Measures (SPS Agreement), is to safeguard world trade by publishing health standards for international trade in animals and animal products. The main normative works produced by the OIE for aquatic animals are the *Aquatic Animal Health Code* and the *Manual of Diagnostic Tests for Aquatic Animals*. They provide a range of tools that assist Member Countries in preventing and controlling aquatic animal diseases. General (i.e., not disease-specific) tools range from recommendations on preventative approaches such as import risk analysies, through guidelines for contingency plans as part of the preparedness and response arrangements of a country, to recommendations on post-incident activities such as fallowing. While the disease-specific chapters of the *Aquatic Code* currently focus on uniform, targeted surveillance requirements for recognition of freedom from infection to underpin health certification prior to trade, future editions of the *Aquatic Code* will provide disease-specific requirements for surveillance and monitoring to allow more flexibility for declaration of freedom from infection with a listed disease. In the future, the *Aquatic Code* will also list commodities that can be traded "safely" without disease-specific restrictions, regardless of the status of the exporting country for the particular disease. The *Aquatic Code* will suggest disease-specific risk management measures for commodities.

Eva-Maria Bernoth. E-mail: eva-maria.bernoth@daff.gov.au

Introduction

The OIE (Office International des Épizooties; World Organisation for Animal Health) is an intergovernmental organization, created in 1924. In March 2004, the OIE totaled 166 Member Countries.

The main objectives of the OIE are

- to ensure transparency in the global animal disease situation;
- to collect, analyze, and disseminate veterinary scientific information;
- to provide expertise and encourage international solidarity in the control of animal diseases;
- within its mandate under the World Trade Organization (WTO) Agreement on the Application of Sanitary and Phytosanitary Measures (SPS Agreement [http://www.wto.org/english/tratop_e/sps_e/spsagr_e.htm]) to safeguard world trade by publishing health standards for international trade in animals and animal products;
- to improve the legal framework and resources of National Veterinary Services; and
- to provide a better guarantee of the safety of food of animal origin and to promote animal welfare through a science-based approach.

The OIE is placed under the authority and control of an International Committee consisting of Delegates designated by the governments of Member Countries. The OIE manages its day-to-day operation through a Central Bureau, situated in Paris, France, placed under the responsibility of a Director General elected by the International Committee.

OIE standards

The OIE develops normative documents relating to rules that Member Countries can use to protect themselves from diseases without setting up unjustified sanitary barriers. The main normative works produced by the OIE for aquatic animals are the *Aquatic Animal Health Code* (the *Aquatic Code*, OIE 2004) and the *Manual of Diagnostic Tests for Aquatic Animals* (the *Aquatic Manual*, OIE 2003).

The aquatic standards are prepared by one of the four elected Specialist Commissions of the OIE, i.e., the Aquatic Animal Health Standards Commission (in brief, Aquatic Animals Commission) with the assistance of internationally renowned experts. The views of the Delegates of Member Countries are systematically sought through the circulation of draft and revised texts.

The Aquatic Animals Commission also collaborates closely with the OIE Terrestrial Animal Health Standards Commission on issues needing a harmonized approach, and with the Biological Standards and Scientific Commissions to ensure that the Aquatic Animals Commission is using the latest scientific information in its work. The OIE International Committee, the general assembly of all Delegates of OIE Member Countries, which constitutes the highest decision-making body of the organization, finally adopts the standards.

The value of the OIE Standards is twofold: (a) the measures published in it are the result of consensus among the veterinary authorities of OIE Member Countries and (b) they constitute a reference within the WTO SPS Agreement as an international standard for animal health and zoonoses.

A new edition of the *Aquatic Code* is published annually. While the *Aquatic Manual* is updated annually, a new edition is produced only every third year. The latest editions of both documents are available online free of charge at the OIE website (www.oie.int).

In the following text, some terms are italicized. This indicates that they are used *sensu stricto*, i.e., in the way that OIE defines them. Where considered crucial to the understanding of this chapter, the exact definitions are provided at the end of this chapter. For other italicized terms, the reader is referred to the 7th edition of the *Aquatic Code* (OIE 2004).

Prevention and control of aquatic animal diseases

The aim of the *Aquatic Code* is to assure the sanitary safety of international trade in aquatic animals (fish, molluscs, and crustaceans) and their products. This is achieved through the detailing of health measures to be used by the *Competent Authorities*[1] of importing and exporting countries to avoid the transfer of agents pathogenic for animals or humans, while avoiding unjustified sanitary barriers.

Provisions in the current editions of the Aquatic Code and Manual for disease prevention and control

The current edition of the *Aquatic Code* includes a range of general, i.e., not disease-specific, provisions that Member Countries can adopt to prevent and control aquatic animal disease. For example, Part 1 of the *Aquatic Code* provides ethical rules for international trade and model aquatic animal health certificates (Section 1.3 in the *Aquatic Code* and Appendices in Part 6). It specifies the rules for disease notification (Section 1.2), including those for new and *emerging diseases*[2]. It outlines the principles of import risk analysis (IRA) (Section 1.4), which includes guidelines for IRAs and a chapter on zoning. There are also guidelines for disease contingency planning (Section 1.6) and fallowing in aquaculture (Section 1.7). Section 1.5 provides standards on import and export procedures. Appendices in Part 5 of the *Aquatic Code* provide information on blood sampling and vaccination and on inactivation of pathogens.

The *Aquatic Manual* contains general requirements for surveillance for recognition of freedom from infection (Chapter 1.1.4) and methods for disinfection of aquaculture establishments (Chapter 1.1.5).

The disease-specific chapters of the *Aquatic Code* (Parts 2 to 4) currently focus on achieving free status regarding the specific disease, and the provisions for achieving free status are solely based on targeted surveillance. For international trade, the status (free or not free) of a country regarding a specific disease is to be documented on an aquatic animal health certificate (models are provided in Part 6 of the *Aquatic Code*) that refers back to the diagnostic and screening methods detailed in the matching disease-specific chapter in the *Aquatic Manual*.

Future editions of the Aquatic Code and Manual and their importance for disease prevention and control

It is important to understand the principal drivers behind the work of the OIE and its Specialist Commissions. These drivers include the need to develop standards that are globally applicable, the need to base standards on science, and the need to harmonize approaches between aquatics and terrestrials.

From a scientific standpoint, there is the need to revise substantially the individual disease chapters of the *Aquatic Code* to take into account the new requirements for surveillance regarding declaration of freedom from infection.

As part of the harmonization with the approaches presented in the *Terrestrial Code*, the new disease chapters for the *Aquatic Code* will introduce, where possible, the concept of "safe commodities" for specific diseases by identifying those commodities for which *Competent Authorities* should authorize trade without restrictions relating to the disease, and regardless of the status of the exporting country regarding the disease in question. Introducing risk management measures that reduce the disease-associated risk of trade in commodities should increase the relevance of chapters to OIE Member Countries.

Declaration of freedom from infection

Chapter 1.1.4 of the *Aquatic Manual* contains general requirements for surveillance for declaration of freedom from infection with a *listed disease*[3]. These requirements differ depending on the previous infection status and take into account, for example, historical freedom and absence of *susceptible species*[4]. Where targeted surveillance is necessary, it needs to be underpinned with scientifically based, disease-specific surveys. This constitutes a graded, risk-based approach. For example, where there are no susceptible species, there is no need for targeted surveillance, but *basic biosecurity conditions* need to be in place.

The following new definitions provide some detail on this approach:

Basic biosecurity conditions are a set of conditions applying to a particular *disease* and a particular *zone* or country, required to ensure adequate disease security, such as:

- the *disease*[5], including suspicion of the *disease*, is compulsorily notifiable to the *Competent Authority*;
- an *early detection system* is in place within the *zone* or country; and
- import requirements to prevent the introduction of *disease* into the country or *zone*, as outlined in the *Aquatic Code*, are in place.

An *early detection system* is an efficient system for ensuring rapid recognition of signs that are suspicious of a *listed disease*, or an *emerging disease* situation, or unexplained mortality, in *aquatic animals*[6] in an *aquaculture establishment* or in the wild, and the rapid communication of the event to the *Competent Authority*, with the aim of activating diagnostic investigation with minimal delay. Such a system will include the following characteristics:

1. Broad awareness, e.g., among the personnel employed at *aquaculture establishments* or involved in *processing*, of the characteristic signs of the *listed diseases* and *emerging diseases*.
2. Veterinarians or aquatic animal health specialists trained in recognizing and reporting suspicious disease occurrence.
3. Ability of the *Competent Authority* to undertake rapid and effective disease investigation.
4. Access by the *Competent Authority* to laboratories with the facilities for diagnosing and differentiating *listed* and *emerging diseases*.

Where targeted surveillance is required, the survey design including sample sizes, should take into account population specifics, disease specifics, design prevalence, and test characteristics. This is a huge step forward from the previous "one-size-fits-all" approach of targeted surveillance of 150/60/30 animals, but it still needs to be "translated" into the disease-specific chapters of the *Aquatic Code* and *Manual*.

Safe commodities

As yet, there is no definition in the *Aquatic Code* for "safe commodities". "Safe commodities" relate to a specific disease. Conceptually, they are those commodities for which *Competent Authorities* should authorize trade without restrictions relating to the disease, and regardless of the exporting country's status regarding the disease in question. This approach would also clarify concerns raised previously regarding the different levels of risk posed by trade in susceptible, carrier, and vector species, and the movement of aquatic animals or eggs or gametes from an infected *aquaculture establishment* or *zone*, by identifying the different risk levels of such commodities.

The new chapters are also to provide guidance on disease-specific risk management measures to manage the risk associated with the importation of certain commodities. The Aquatic Animals Commission will, over the next years and in consultation with the Terrestrial Animal Health Standards Commission, develop a template on which to base individual disease chapters for the *Aquatic Code*. These chapters will be submitted for progressive adoption by the International Committee, and will serve as models for the development of all disease chapters of the *Aquatic Code*, based on the work of international experts including experts from OIE Reference Laboratories.

Conclusion

The OIE *Aquatic Code* provides a range of tools that assist Member Countries in preventing and controlling aquatic animal diseases. General (i.e., not disease-specific) tools range from recommendations on preventative approaches, such as IRAs, through guidelines for contingency plans as part of the preparedness and response arrangements of a country, to recommendations on post-incident activities such as fallowing. While the disease-specific chapters of the *Aquatic Code* currently focus on uniform, targeted surveillance for recognition of freedom from infection to underpin health certification prior to trade, future editions of the *Aquatic Code* will provide disease-specific requirements for surveillance and monitoring to allow more flexibility for declaration of freedom from infection with a listed disease. In the future, the *Aquatic Code* will also list commodities that can be traded safely without disease-specific restrictions and regardless of the status of the exporting country for the particular disease, and it will suggest disease-specific risk management measures for commodities.

References

OIE (Office International des Epizooties). 2003. *Manual of Diagnostic Tests for Aquatic Animals*, 3rd edition. Office International des Epizooties, Paris, France. 358 pp.

OIE (Office International des Epizooties). 2004. *Aquatic Animal Health Code*, 7th edition. Office International des Epizooties, Paris, France. 167 pp.

Definitions

Definitions for the following terms are from the 7th edition of the *Aquatic Code* (OIE 2004).

1. *Competent Authority*: The National Veterinary Services, or other Authority of a Member Country, having the responsibility and competence for ensuring or supervising the implementation of the aquatic animal health measures recommended in this *Aquatic Code*.
2. *Emerging disease*: A newly recognised serious disease, the cause of which may or may not yet be established, which has the potential to spread within and between populations, for example by way of trade in *aquatic animals* and/or *aquatic animal products*.
3. *Diseases listed by the OIE*: *Diseases* that fulfill the criteria outlined in Chapter 1.1.2 of the OIE *Aquatic Code*.
4. *Susceptible species*: A species of *aquatic animal* in which a *disease agent* can multiply or otherwise develop.
5. *Disease*: Clinical or nonclinical infection with one or more of the aetiological agents of the *diseases* listed in this *Aquatic Code*.
6. *Aquatic animals*: All life stages (including *eggs* and *gametes*) of fish, molluscs, and crustaceans originating from *aquaculture establishments* or removed from the wild, for farming purposes, for release into the aquatic environment or for human consumption.

Chapter 2

Biosecurity in Aquaculture: International Agreements and Instruments, their Compliance, Prospects, and Challenges for Developing Countries

Rohana P. Subasinghe and Melba G. Bondad-Reantaso

Abstract

Aquaculture is the fastest growing food producing sector in the world. Besides providing food, it generates employment and income, and supports livelihoods of many millions of people all over the world. Diseases and epizootics are considered to be major concerns for increasing production through aquaculture and for the sectoral development. Most disease threats have so far resulted from unregulated movement of live aquatic animals and associated introductions and/or transfers of pathogens. Over the years, many attempts have been made to prevent and control disease emergencies in aquaculture, both with documented successes and failures. Controlling diseases in small-scale production systems, which are the core of most global production, is particularly challenging as implementation of control measures is difficult, and resources for prevention are limited. It has been realized that the best approach to managing aquatic animal health is to improve biosecurity at all levels. Biosecurity provides a strategic framework and integrated approach to assess and manage the risks that threaten food safety, animal life and health, plant life and health, and associated environmental perils.

There are international instruments for controlling the spread of pathogens, thus improving biosecurity in farming systems. Compliance with these standards, however, is not an easy task for many developing countries. This chapter describes the role of biosecurity for reducing disease risks in aquaculture and the opportunities and challenges for developing countries, through an example from a recent study conducted in controlling disease in shrimp aquaculture in India.

Rohana P. Subasinghe, corresponding author. E-mail: rohana.subasinghe@fao.org

Introduction

Health maintenance in aquaculture is now considered to be one of the most important aspects of aquaculture development and management. Over the years, serious and significant damage to the sector, in different parts of the world, has caused considerable economic damage. The most appropriate explanation of the cause is lack of biosecurity. Realization of the importance of keeping pathogens away from farms made biosecurity of paramount importance for aquatic animal health management.

Biosecurity and agriculture

Biosecurity is a relatively new concept and a term that is evolving as usage varies among countries with different specialist groups using it in different ways. *Biosecurity* broadly describes the process and objective of managing biological risks associated with food and agriculture in a holistic manner.* *Biosecurity* measures in agriculture are needed:

- to protect agricultural production systems, and those dependent on these systems. Producers and others dependent on agriculture can see their livelihood destroyed by animal and plant pests and disease or damage to the environment, such as impacts resulting from invasive alien species;
- to protect human health and consumer confidence in agricultural products. *Biosecurity* measures are essential to protect consumers (who are particularly vulnerable) who can be exposed to severe health risks; and
- to protect the environment and promote sustainable production. Public awareness of environmental issues and human dependence on biodiversity has resulted in numerous commitments to achieving sustainable development, and achieving these will require an effective approach to *biosecurity*.

Biosecurity is a strategic and integrated approach that encompasses the policy and regulatory frameworks (including instruments and activities) that analyze and manage risks in the sectors of food safety, animal life and health, and plant life and health, including associated environmental risk. *Biosecurity* covers the introduction of plant pests, animal pests and diseases, and zoonoses; the introduction and release of genetically modified organisms (GMOs) and their products; and the introduction and management of invasive alien species and genotypes. *Biosecurity* is a holistic concept of direct relevance to the sustainability of agriculture, food safety, and the protection of the environment, including biodiversity.

The issues encompassed in *biosecurity* have traditionally been dealt with in a sectoral manner by means of food safety laws and animal and plant quarantine and pesticide regulations. Implementation of such laws and regulations has also traditionally been sectoral. To respond to emerging issues of biosafety, and to control the introduction and management of invasive alien species into the environment, a growing number of issues need to be addressed. This results in costly regulatory systems that require high investment and recurrent costs (infrastructure and human resources).

* With "agriculture," biosecurity is used in its broadest sense to include agronomy, livestock, forestry, fisheries, and related environmental aspects.

Biosecurity and aquaculture

Aquaculture is the fastest growing food-producing sector in the world. A high proportion (over 90%) of this production originates in the developing world. In contrast to terrestrial farming systems, where the bulk of global production is based on a limited number of animal and plant species, the aquaculture sector comprises over 230 different species. This large number of species cultivated reflects the diversity of the sector, including the range and complexity of environments used, the different production systems and intensity of practice, and the type of management used. According to latest Food and Agriculture Organization of the United Nations (FAO) statistics, the contribution of aquaculture to global supplies of fish, crustaceans, and molluscs increased from 3.9% of total production by weight in 1970 to 29.9% in 2002. Aquaculture continues to grow more rapidly than all other animal food producing sectors. Worldwide, the sector has grown at an average rate of 8.9% per year, since 1970, compared to only 1.2% for capture fisheries and 2.8% for terrestrial farmed meat production systems over the same period. Production from aquaculture has greatly outpaced population growth, with per capita supply from aquaculture increasing from 0.7 kg in 1970 to 6.4 kg in 2002, an average annual growth rate of 7.2%.

Alien aquatic species and genotypes (also known as introduced species and genetically altered species) have a major role in increasing production. While alien species can pose a negative threat to the aquatic biodiversity and socio-economic well-being of a nation, there are also recognizable social and economic benefits from the introduction and farming of some alien aquatic species. About 17% of the world's finfish production results from alien species. Asia produces more of the African cichlid tilapia (>700,000 tons) than Africa itself (39,245 tons). In Chile, introduced salmonids provide over 20% of the world's farmed salmon, in an industry directly employing more than 30,000 people. The issue is neither to ban alien species, nor to abandon the regulation of their movement, but to assess the risks and, if appropriate, develop and implement plans for their responsible use.

Although aquaculture is the fastest growing food-production sector, diseases are a primary constraint to the growth of aquaculture in many parts of the world. A multitude of factors has contributed to the health problems currently faced by aquaculture. Over the past three decades, aquaculture has expanded, intensified, and diversified, based heavily on movements of live aquatic animals and animal products (broodstock, seed, and feed). Changing circumstances and perspectives, and especially, world trade liberalization have triggered this trend. New outlooks and directions have accelerated the accidental spread and incursion of diseases into new populations and geographic regions, for example, through movements of hatchery produced stocks, new species for culture, and enhancement and development of the ornamental fish trade.

Although translocation of pathogens and diseases with movements of their hosts is not a new phenomenon, it has only recently gained focused attention in many regions. Advances in live aquatic animal trade, facilitated by improved transportation efficiency, are now recognized as having played a pivotal role in the introduction and spread of pathogens and diseases into many aquaculture systems, causing *biosecurity* threats to the sector and the production systems. Factors such as food security, protection of the natural environment, biodiversity conservation, societal demands for healthy products, and the general socio-economic development and well-being of a nation have driven the improvement of *biosecurity* practices.

In aquaculture, *biosecurity* is a collective term that refers to the concept of applying appropriate measures (e.g., proactive disease risk analysis) to reduce the probability of a biological organism or agent spreading to an individual, population, or ecosystem, and to mitigate the adverse impact that may result (Arthur et al. 2004). This analysis is done in a way that incorporates the best information available on aspects of husbandry, epidemiology, and sound science. The goal can be thought of as minimizing both exposure to and economic loss from disease-related causes, physico-chemical impacts, ecological impacts, nutritional parameters, predation, and more. *Biosecurity* stresses the development of a series of protocols to respond to disease exposure risks that have been assessed through a careful on-site audit, usually by an aquatic animal veterinarian or a qualified aquatic animal health expert.

Biosecurity standards

Food and agriculture markets are increasingly becoming global as consumers demand a diversity of products, all year round. People consuming food grown elsewhere in the world require trust that those products are healthy, of good quality, and safe to eat, and the *biosecurity* systems in place in producing and importing countries are adequate. Common product standards would thus provide not only a basis for trade between countries, but also the basis for improved confidence and trust between producers and consumers. As confidence between trading partners builds through experience, the rate of product testing is reduced and transaction costs go down. International movement of animals and plants associated with food or food production sectors are increasing. All these cause risks to humans and the environment. The role of agreed international standards is therefore of great economic and ecological importance.

Harmonization of standards and procedures for improving *biosecurity* is important for addressing hazards in food safety, particularly when applying the whole food chain approach. It is also important for better quality and safety, especially for trade-driven comparability of products, for responding to expanding risks resulting from increased trade and travel, and to cope with advances in modern biotechnology and information technology.

Internationally recognized treaties have recently been established to address the issue. Some of these agreements are binding and some are non-binding.

International measures

The Aquatic Animal Health Code

International *biosecurity* standards for the movement of aquatic animals and their products have been developed by the World Organisation for Animal Health (Office International des Epizooties, OIE). The diseases listed by the OIE reflect aquatic animal species that are important to aquaculture and trade. Diseases are listed based on their characteristics in terms of consequence, spread, and diagnosis. Although the movement of live brood stock and genetic material is the main concern, movement of products has also recently been considered.

The current OIE Aquatic Animal Health Code (the Aquatic Code; OIE 2004) provides health standards for the movement of live aquatic animals and their genetic material diseases listed by the OIE. The Aquatic Code also contains recommendations for dead, uneviscerated fish and dead crustaceans with respect to the listed diseases. Member countries of the OIE are obliged to report disease occurrences to the international community through the OIE. Disease reporting is intended to assist in minimizing disease risks.

The Agreement on the Application of Sanitary and Phytosanitary Measures

The World Trade Organization (WTO) Agreement on the Application of Sanitary and Phytosanitary Measures (SPS Agreement) provides a basic right to WTO member countries to take necessary measures to protect human, animal, or plant life or health (WTO 1994). With this right, come certain obligations including one that such protective measures must be based on a risk assessment or conform to an international standard. In the case of aquatic animal health, the measures in the Aquatic Code are the relevant international standards.

Members of the WTO are also able to take provisional measures in cases where relevant scientific evidence is insufficient for the risk assessment. This is often the situation in aquatic disease emergencies while the disease agent is being identified, the extent of its spread is being determined, the effectiveness of control measures are being assessed, and trace back and trace forward investigations are continuing. WTO members adopting provisional measures must consider the available pertinent information, including international standards, seek further information to assess the risk, and review the measure in a timely manner. Individual aquaculture producers can practice on-farm biosecurity to help minimize losses and facilitate a faster return to market.

International standards for food safety, plant health, and animal health

The Codex Alimentarius Commission (Codex), the International Plant Protection Convention (IPPC), and the OIE provide international standards for food safety, plant health, and animal health, respectively. A further relevant instrument (not yet entered into force) is the Cartagena protocol (SCBD 2000), which applies to the transboundary movement, transit, handling, and use of living genetically modified organisms (LMOs). Guidelines on the management of invasive alien species (SCBD 2000) have been developed under the Convention on Biological Diversity (CBD). This group of international agreements, organizations, and programs are part of a loose international framework for *biosecurity*, and reflect the historically sectoral approach to regulation in this area.

The international movement of eggs and gametes is infrequent (particularly in Asia). This method, however, is recommended by the international codes of practice for species introductions (e.g., the International Council for the Exploration of the Sea [ICES] and the European Inland Fisheries Advisory Commission [EIFAC]), as it generally involves a lower risk of pathogen transfer (see Turner 1988; ICES 2003).

Opportunities and challenges for developing countries

Many developed countries have been able to respond adequately in improving *biosecurity* practices. Developing countries are facing problems. Convergence or harmonization within and between countries, however, is beginning to occur, at least in some countries. Response to these new challenges has to date been piecemeal, particularly in institutional terms. Regulatory costs are very high. There are growing signs of a cross-sectoral approach to regulation.

Technical details of farm level *biosecurity* and health management in shrimp aquaculture and biosecurity measures in a specific pathogen free facility are available (see for example,

Lotz 1997; Chanratchakool et al. 1998; Fegan and Clifford 2001; Fegan et al. 2001). One of the greatest challenges lies in responsibilities commonly distributed among a number of institutions, to ensure that functions are performed effectively (control) and efficiently (costs). Crucial elements in this process include cross-institutional cooperation and commitment in defining tasks, objectives, and priorities, and agreement on division of labor and resources. This is extremely difficult in many developing countries, as most governments just do not have adequate resources or the capacity to deal with the logistic requirements of *biosecurity* programs. In achieving aquaculture *biosecurity*, the most difficult problem to deal with is the large numbers of small farms, particularly in Asia. Opportunities, however, exist in empowering the farmers, mainly through establishing self-regulatory processors and mechanisms.

Experiences with small-scale shrimp aquaculture

A practical example of a biosecurity program is demonstrated by a shrimp disease control project in southern India implemented in 2000 by the Marine Products Export Development Authority (MPEDA) of India, Ministry of Commerce and Industry, with technical assistance from the Network of Aquaculture Centres in Asia–Pacific (NACA) (Padiyar et al. 2003).

The initial study, in 2000, in West Godavari and Nellore districts of the State of Andhra Pradesh, where more than 70% of the Indian shrimp production originates, used an epidemiological approach to identify the key risk factors for white spot disease (WSD) and to better understand the role of these factors in disease outbreaks and low pond production. The outcomes of this study led to the development of better management practices (BMPs) to reduce the identified risks, followed by wide consultation with farmers and other agencies to gather consensus on the study findings and their practical application to improve performance of shrimp farming systems of Andhra Pradesh. The BMPs included three main management strategies focusing on: (a) pond bottom preparation and water management prior to stocking, (b) seed selection and stocking, and (c) post-stocking management. On-farm testing of BMPs followed, using a few selected farms. The process was monitored and evaluated to understand benefits and constraints. Information on risk management strategies was widely disseminated to farmers. Improved pond level risk management practices reduced incidence of disease and led to improvements in profits and productivity. In demonstration farms, returns shifted from a loss in 80% of ponds in 2001 to a profit in 80% of ponds in 2002.

Following this success, in 2003, village demonstrations were expanded to 256 ponds covering over 125 ha of land belonging to 98 farmers. The farmers voluntarily worked with the study team and formed an "Aquaclub" to implement the BMPs through this local networking approach. The "Aquaclub" met regularly, promoted widespread adoption of BMPs among its members, generated interest among neighboring villages, and most importantly, gained significant benefits from this cooperative approach.

The details of the BMPs developed and implemented from the above project are presented below.

a. Pond bottom preparation and water management prior to stocking.
   - Sludge removal and disposal away from the pond site.
   - Plowing on wet soil if the sludge has not been removed completely.
   - Water filtration using twin bag filters of 300 μm mesh size.
   - Water depth of at least 80 cm at the shallowest part of pond.
   - Water conditioning for 10–15 days before stocking.

b. Seed selection and stocking.
   - Uniform size and color post-larvae (PLs), actively swimming against the water current.
   - Nested polymerase chain reaction negative PLs for WSD (using batches of 59 PLs pooled together). If the test turns negative, it indicates that the prevalence of WSD infected PLs is less than 5% in that population at 95% confidence.
   - Weak PL elimination before stocking using formalin (100 ppm) stress for 15–20 minutes in continuously aerated water.
   - On-farm nursery rearing of PLs for 15–20 days.
   - Stocking during the first week of February to the second week of March.
   - Stocking into green water and avoiding transparent water during stocking.

c. Post stocking management.
   - Use of water reservoirs, and 10–15 days aging before use in grow out ponds.
   - Regular use of agricultural lime, especially after water exchange and rain.
   - No use of any harmful/banned chemicals.
   - Use of feed check trays to ensure feeding based on shrimp demand.
   - Feeding across the pond using boat/floating device to avoid local waste accumulation.
   - Regular removal of benthic algae.
   - Water exchanges only during critical periods.
   - Weekly checking of pond bottom mud for blackish organic waste accumulation and unpleasant odor.
   - Regular shrimp health checks, and weekly health and growth monitoring using a cast net.
   - Removal and safe disposal of sick or dead shrimp.
   - Emergency harvesting after proper decision-making.
   - No draining or abandoning of disease-affected stocks.

The farm level *biosecurity* experience in India suggests a need to carefully develop situation-specific BMPs with farmers (based on general BMP principles) tailored to the farming systems (based on stocking densities, ability to maintain water reservoirs, source, water quality, etc.) and investment capacity of individual farmers.

Educating farmers about the risks, engaging them in assessing and managing the risks through a cooperative approach via local networking and self-help programs are important components of a biosecurity program. Because of the demonstrated benefit to farmers, the work has now been extended to several other districts in Andhra Pradesh. The FAO has provided technical and financial assistance for expanding and widely applying the concept and developing more situation-specific BMPs. This follow-up project now addresses the issue of application of BMPs and the management of clusters of shrimp farms and farmers—cluster management in small-scale shrimp aquaculture—taking into consideration the lessons learned and addressing broader environmental, social, and economic sustainability of the sector, based on an epidemiological approach to health management.

Acknowledgments

The authors wish to acknowledge MPEDA and NACA for providing permission to use the experimental data. Special appreciation goes to Mr. Arun Padiyar, Dr. Michael Phillips,

Mr. Mongkhon Primphon, Dr. C.V. Mohan, Mr. Vishnu Bhat, Mr. V.S. VS Rao, and Mr. G. Ravi for their untiring work, which led to the success of this study.

References

Arthur, J.R., M.G. Bondad-Reantaso, F.C. Baldock, C.J. Rodgers, and B.F. Edgerton. 2004. *Manual on Risk Analysis for the Safe Movement of Aquatic Animals (FWG/01/2002).* APEC/DoF/NACA/FAO, Bangkok, Thailand. 59 pp.

Chanratchakool, P., J.F. Turnbull, S.J. Funge-Smith, I.H. MacRae, and C. Limsuan. 1998. *Health Management in Shrimp Ponds.* Aquatic Animal Health Research Institute, Department of Fisheries, Kasetsart University Campus, Jatujak, Bangkok, Thailand. 152 pp.

FAO (Food and Agriculture Organization of the United Nations). 2003. *Health Management and Biosecurity Maintenance in White Shrimp (Penaeus vannamei) Hatcheries in Latin America.* FAO Fisheries Technical Paper No. 450. FAO, Rome, Italy. 58 pp.

Fegan, D.F., J.R. Arthur, R.P. Subasinghe, M.B. Reantaso, V. Alday de Graindorge, and M.J. Phillips. 2001. Consultant Report: A review of trans-boundary aquatic animal pathogen introductions and transfers. Pages 132–174 *in APEC/FAO/NACA/SEMARNAP. Trans-boundary Aquatic Animal Pathogen Transfer and the Development of Harmonized Standards on Aquaculture Health Management.* Report of the joint APEC/FAO/NACA/SEMARNAP Workshop, Puerto Vallarta, Jalisco, Mexico, 24–28 July 2000. Network of Aquaculture Centres in Asia–Pacific, Bangkok, Thailand.

Fegan, D.F. and H.C. Clifford III. 2001. Health management for viral disease in shrimp farms. Pages 168–198 *in* C.L. Browdy and D.E. Jory, editors. *The New Wave: Proceedings of the Special Session on Sustainable Shrimp Farming.* The World Aquaculture Society, Baton Rouge, LA.

ICES (International Council for the Exploration of the Sea). 2003. *ICES Code of Practice on the Introductions and Transfers of Marine Organisms 2003.* International Council for the Exploration of the Sea, Copenhagen, Denmark. 28 pp. On-line version, http://www.ices.dk/reports/general/2003/Codemarineintroductions2003.pdf

Lotz, J.M. 1997. Disease control and pathogen status assurance in an SPF-based shrimp aquaculture industry, with particular reference to the United States. Pages 243–254 *in* T.W. Flegel and I.H. MacRae, editors. *Diseases in Asian Aquaculture III.* Fish Health Section, Asian Fisheries Society, Manila, Philippines.

OIE (World Organisation for Animal Health). 2004. *International Aquatic Animal Health Code,* 7th edition. World Organisation for Animal Health (OIE), Paris, France. On-line version, http://www.oie.int/eng/normes/fcode/A_summry.htm

Padiyar, P.A., M.J. Phillips, M. Primphon, C.V. Mohan, B.V. Bhat, V.S. Rao, and G. Ravi. Extension in shrimp health management: experiences from an MPEDA/NACA program in Andhra Pradesh, India. *Aquaculture Asia,* July–September 2003, 7–13.

SCBD (Secretariat of the Convention on Biological Diversity). 2000. *Cartagena Protocol on Biosafety to the Convention on Biological Diversity: Text and Annexes.* Secretariat of the Convention on Biological Diversity, Montreal, Quebec, Canada. 30 pp. On-line version, http://www.biodiv.org/biosafety/protocol.asp

Turner, G.E., editor. 1988. *Codes of Practice and Manual of Procedures for Consideration of Introductions and Transfers of Marine and Freshwater Organisms.* EIFAC Occasional Paper No. 23. European Inland Fisheries Advisory Commission, FAO, Rome, Italy. 44 p.

WTO (World Trade Organization). 1994. Agreement on the Application of Sanitary and Phytosanitary Measures. Pages 69–84 *in The Results of the Uruguay Round of Multilateral Trade Negotiations: The Legal Texts.* General Agreement on Tariffs and Trade (GATT), World Trade Organization, Geneva, Switzerland.

Chapter 3

Regional Approach to Aquatic Animal Health Management—Views and Programs of the Network of Aquaculture Centres in Asia–Pacific

C.V. Mohan and Melba G. Bondad-Reantaso

Abstract

The Network of Aquaculture Centres in Asia–Pacific (NACA), an inter-governmental organization with 16 member countries and five participating governments in the Asia–Pacific region, seeks to promote rural development through sustainable aquaculture and responsible trade in aquaculture products. Aquaculture in the region is expanding, diversifying, and intensifying to become a major food-producing sector. The spread of aquatic animal pathogens has directly led to serious disease outbreaks in the region, impacting aquaculture productivity, livelihoods, trade, and national economies. Such problems have also indirectly impacted the trade of aquatic animal products within Asia and between Asia and major trading partners.

Addressing aquatic animal health issues through proactive cooperation is one of the key program areas of NACA, with the purpose of assisting member governments to "reduce the risks of aquatic animal diseases impacting the livelihoods of aquaculture farmers, national economies, trade, environment, and human health." The NACA implements its programs throughout the region in partnership with governments, industry, non-governmental organizations, donors, and development agencies. With the Food and Agriculture Organization of the United Nations (FAO), the World Organisation for Animal Health (Office International des Epizooties, OIE), and with regional and international expertise, guiding principles for responsible movement of aquatic animals and aquatic animal health management have been established. The guiding principles in the "Asia Regional Technical Guidelines on Health Management and the Responsible Movement of Live Aquatic Animals," were adopted by 21 governments in the Asian region, in 2000.

The various components identified in the Technical Guidelines are now the main focus of NACA's Regional Aquatic Animal Health Program. This chapter will provide a brief insight of the important aquatic animal health issues in the region, and will highlight some of the key regional activities and accomplishments under NACA's Regional Aquatic Animal Health Program.

C.V. Mohan, corresponding author. E-mail: mohan@enaca.org

Introduction

Diseases are one of the major bottlenecks for the development of the aquaculture sector in the Asia–Pacific region. Trans-boundary movement of live aquatic animals in the region is one of the principal reasons for increased occurrence and spread of several serious diseases (Subasinghe et al. 2001; Bondad-Reantaso 2001a, 2004a). Examples of diseases and pathogens introduced to new areas and hosts leading to serious consequences in the Asia–Pacific region include the epizootic ulcerative syndrome (EUS) in fresh and brackish water fishes, white spot syndrome virus (WSSV) and Taura syndrome virus (TSV) in cultured shrimp, and viral encephalopathy and retinopathy (VER) in grouper. Continued mass mortalities of common carp (*Cyprinus carpio* L.) and koi (*C. carpio*) in Indonesia since June 2002, and the confirmed outbreak of koi herpes virus (KHV) in Japan (NACA/FAO 2004) are sad reminders of the dangers associated with trans-boundary spread of pathogens. The spread of aquatic animal pathogens has directly led to serious disease outbreaks in Asia. Careful examination of the history and spread of these diseases in the region indicate how irresponsible or ill-considered movements of live animals can impact aquaculture and wild fisheries resources.

Sound health management protocols incorporating principles of biosecurity, at the pond, farm, national, and regional levels, is increasingly becoming crucial for ensuring successful and sustainable aquaculture. Current efforts under the Regional Aquatic Animal Health Program of the Network of Aquaculture Centres in Asia–Pacific (NACA), in cooperation with the constituent member governments, and regional and international partners in development (e.g., the Aquatic Animal Health Research Institute [AAHRI]; the Australian Centre for International Agricultural Research [ACIAR]; the Asia–Pacific Economic Cooperation [APEC]; the Association of Southeast Asian Nations [ASEAN]; the Commonwealth Scientific and Industrial Research Organization [CSIRO], in Australia; the Australian Agency for International Aid [AusAID]; the FAO; the OIE; the Mekong River Commission [MRC]; and the Southeast Asian Fisheries Development Center [SEAFDEC]) are geared towards promoting science-based, yet practical health management strategies in the region.

Diseases of concern to the Asia–Pacific region

Some of the most serious problems faced by the aquaculture sector in the Asia–Pacific region are those pathogens and diseases introduced and spread through movements of hatchery produced stocks, new species for aquaculture, and the ornamental fish trade. Socio-economic and other impacts of diseases in selected Asian countries are comprehensively reviewed by Subasinghe et al. (2001) and Bondad-Reantaso (2004a). Israngkura and Sae-Hae (2002) estimated that combined losses from shrimp diseases, at the global level from 11 countries for the period 1987–1994, were U.S.$ 3 billion. More recent examples of economic losses due to spread of aquatic animal diseases include the following: (a) carp mortalities in Indonesia, with estimated losses of 50 billion Indonesian rupiahs, approximately U.S.$ 5.5 million (NACA /ACIAR 2002); (b) losses due to KHV in Japan, estimated to be 150 million yen, approximately U.S.$ 1.4 million (ISID 2003a); and (c) abalone mortalities

Table 3.1 Occurrence (+) of important finfish and crustacean trans-boundary diseases in Asia–Pacific, according to the NACA/FAO/OIE regional Quarterly Aquatic Animal Disease (QAAD) reporting system

	Disease					
Country	EUS	VER	Iridoviral disease	Infection with KHV	White spot disease	Taura syndrome
Australia	+	+				
Bangladesh	+				+	
Cambodia	+				+	
PR China					+	+
DPR Korea (North Korea)						
Hong Kong, China		+	+			
India	+				+	
Indonesia	+	+	+	+	+	+
Iran					+	
Japan	+	+		+	+	
Lao PDR	+					
Malaysia	+	+			+	
Myanmar	+				+	
Nepal	+					
Pakistan	+					
Philippines	+	+			+	
RO Korea (South Korea)		+			+	
Singapore		+	+		+	
Sri Lanka	+				+	
Thailand	+	+			+	+
Vietnam	+	+			+	+

Note: EUS, epizootic ulcerative syndrome; VER, viral encephalopathy and retinopathy; KHV, koi herpes virus.

in Taiwan, estimated to be 400 million Taiwan dollars, approximately U.S.$ 11.4 million (ISID 2003b).

Confirmed reports of important trans-boundary aquatic animal diseases, based on the information published in the NACA / FAO/OIE Quarterly Aquatic Animal Disease (QAAD Asia–Pacific) (1998–2003) reporting system, are provided in Table 3.1. In addition to the OIE-listed and the NACA/FAO/OIE-listed diseases, there are many more diseases of regional and national interests that have impacted Asian aquaculture (Subasinghe et al. 2001; Bondad-Reantaso 2004a), and some are newly emerging in the region. The section below briefly describes some of the most significant diseases occurring in the Asia–Pacific region.

Finfish diseases

Since its first appearance in the early 1980s in Asia, EUS has spread throughout much of Asia–Pacific, and has been reported from 15 countries in the region. While EUS is known by different names, such as mycotic granulomatosis in Japan, red spot disease in Australia, and ulcerative mycosis in the United States, the disease is now largely believed to have a single causative agent, i.e., *Aphanomyces* (*Aphanomyces invadans/piscicida*). The VER causes serious problems to grouper culture in the Asia–Pacific. First reported from Japan in

1991, VER is now widespread occurring in at least 10 countries in the Asia–Pacific region. The mass mortalities of common and koi carps in Indonesia (NACA/ACIAR 2002) and the confirmed KHV outbreaks among cultured carps in Japan (NACA/FAO 2004) are some of the emerging diseases. In recent years, grouper iridoviral disease has also been recognized as increasingly important for the region (Bondad-Reantaso et al. 2001b). Infection with KHV and grouper iridoviral disease are currently not included in the OIE list, but both infections present serious threats to the aquaculture and ornamental industry sectors and trade in the region.

Shrimp diseases

White spot disease caused by WSSV remains the most serious disease affecting 15 of the shrimp producing countries in Asia, and continues to cause serious disease outbreaks in *Penaeus monodon* in many countries of the region (NACA/FAO 2003, 2004). There are reports of WSSV causing mortalities in cultured *Litopenaeus vannamei* in the People's Republic of China (PR China) and Indonesia. Taura syndrome caused by TSV was reported in *L. vannamei* from PR China, Indonesia, and Thailand in 2003 (NACA/FAO 2003, 2004). Introduction of *L. vannamei* is largely believed to be responsible for the introduction of TSV to the Asia–Pacific region. Reports of TSV in native *P. monodon* from Indonesia and PR China are also a cause for concern. Other newly emerging diseases in shrimp aquaculture include infection with Mourilyan virus, a new bunya-related virus affecting penaeid prawns in Australia and possibly elsewhere in the region (Cowley et al. 2002), slow growth syndrome in *P. monodon* (Chayaburakul et al. 2004), and the white tail/body disease in freshwater shrimp *Macrobrachium rosenbergii* (Widada et al. 2004).

Molluscan diseases

Little attention has so far been given to molluscan diseases in the region, although serious losses are known to be occurring. This may indicate the limited diagnostic and technical capacity of molluscan diseases in the region. Of the 35 diseases listed by the OIE, 11 are diseases of molluscs. Some of these pathogens (e.g., *Bonamia exitiosus*, *Haplosporidium nelsoni*, *Marteilia sydneyi*, *Perkinsus olseni*) are known to occur in the region. In addition to the OIE-listed and the NACA/FAO/OIE-listed diseases, there are many more molluscan diseases of regional and national interest (Bondad-Reantaso 2004a). Recent mass mortalities of small abalone (*Haliotis diversicolor*) in Taiwan (ISID 2003b) are of serious concern to the region since Japan, Australia, Republic of Korea (South Korea), and PR China have large abalone industries.

Key NACA regional programs and outputs

The NACA is an inter-governmental organization with 16 member governments (i.e., Australia, Bangladesh, Cambodia, PR China, Hong Kong China, India, Iran, Democratic People's Republic of Korea [North Korea], Malaysia, Myanmar, Nepal, Pakistan, the Philippines, Sri Lanka, Thailand, and Vietnam). Together with a number of actively participating governments including Indonesia, South Korea, Lao People's Democratic

Republic, and Singapore, NACA seeks to promote rural development through sustainable aquaculture and responsible trade in aquaculture products. The mission of NACA is to assist the member governments to improve opportunities for sustainable aquaculture, and to contribute to social and economic development in the Asia–Pacific region. Aquatic animal health management and disease control has been a major component and a priority element of the NACA's Third Five-Year Work Programme (2001–2005). Since 1986, NACA has been actively involved in addressing aquatic animal health issues in the region. Bondad-Reantaso (2001) provided a detailed chronological account of the NACA's Regional Aquatic Animal Health Program. The following section provides brief highlights on some of the major regional approaches and their outputs.

Asia Regional Technical Guidelines on responsible health management

Within Asia, "The Asia Regional Technical Guidelines on Health Management for the Responsible Movement of Live Aquatic Animals" (or, Technical Guidelines) and their associated implementation plan, the Beijing Consensus and Implementation Strategy, provide the basic framework and guidance for national and regional efforts in reducing the risks of diseases due to trans-boundary movement of live aquatic animals, and gives emphasis to the concept of "phased implementation based on national needs" (FAO/NACA 2000). There is strong endorsement by many regional, inter-governmental, and global organizations, and a shared commitment from national governments to support its implementation. The main elements of the Technical Guidelines are guiding principles, pathogens to be considered, disease diagnosis, health certification and quarantine measures, disease zoning, disease surveillance and reporting, contingency planning, import risk analysis (IRA), national strategies and policy frameworks, regional capacity building, and an implementation strategy. The framework provided by the Technical Guidelines is a comprehensive one that includes all major requirements for managing risks associated with the movement of live aquatic animals and trans-boundary pathogens.

The Technical Guidelines were the major output of the regional program requested by 15 Asian governments for FAO assistance and implemented by NACA in 1998 through an FAO Regional Technical Cooperation Program (TCP/RAS 6714 and 9605) project, "Assistance for the Responsible Movement of Live Aquatic Animals in Asia." The regional project was supported by a number of regional and international organizations and agencies. Twenty-one governments/territories in the Asia–Pacific region participated in the project. Bondad-Reantaso (2001) described in detail the 3-year (1998–2001) project development and implementation process. The Technical Guidelines had two companion documents to further support its implementation. These are (a) the Manual of Procedures (FAO/NACA 2001), which contains the background material and detailed technical procedures to assist countries and territories in the Asian region in implementing the Technical Guidelines and (b) the Asia Diagnostic Guide to Aquatic Animal Diseases (Bondad-Reantaso et al. 2001a), which contains comprehensive information for disease diagnosis to support implementation of the Technical Guidelines. All these documents take into full consideration the provisions of the WTO Agreement on the Application of Sanitary and Phytosanitary Measures (WTO-SPS Agreement, WTO 1994), the OIE Aquatic Animal Health Standards (OIE 2003, 2004), as well as Article 9, Aquaculture Development, of the Code of Conduct for Responsible Fisheries (CCRF; FAO 1995).

Current efforts of NACA and its partners are geared towards supporting implementation. Countries who have participated in the regional program are at different stages of development in terms of the National Strategy on Aquatic Animal Health. The National Strategy contains the action plans of governments which form the basis for the implementation of the Technical Guidelines at the national level. There has been considerable progress implementing the Technical Guidelines in several countries in the region (Bondad-Reantaso 2004b). Progress in other countries, however, is rather limited. As implementation of the Technical Guidelines is a long-term process, continuous effort to motivate and support governments in initiating their health management programs is required. Regional workshops, where governments come together and share knowledge and lessons learnt, have proved useful in the past, and should be continued where appropriate to facilitate the process of consensus building and awareness raising, thus generating support for its implementation. Governments tend to pay more attention to their international obligations when trade issues start to affect them, and aquatic animal diseases are becoming a more significant international trade issue. Commitment and willingness on the part of the governments are a primary basis for the implementation of the Technical Guidelines.

Asia–Pacific quarterly aquatic animal disease reporting system

The reporting system for aquatic animal diseases was developed following the recommendations of the NACA/OIE Expert Consultation in 1996 and was eventually integrated into the Regional program. Implementing a regional disease reporting system is one of the key activities of NACA regional programs. The NACA/FAO/OIE quarterly aquatic animal disease (QAAD) reporting system is an example of such cooperation in the Asian region. To date, 22 quarterly issues have been published and widely disseminated in the region (NACA/FAO 2004). The NACA/FAO/OIE disease list includes all diseases listed by OIE, plus diseases of concern to the region. The OIE Aquatic Animal Health Code (OIE 2004) lists 35 diseases of finfish, molluscs, and crustaceans based on three criteria (i.e., consequence, spread, and diagnosis) and thus should be reported to the OIE by member governments. The NACA/FAO/OIE QAAD-Asia–Pacific reporting system lists 44 diseases including those that are non-OIE listed (Table 3.2). The information generated through the regional reporting system provides up-to-date information on important diseases in the Asia–Pacific region, serves as an early warning system for emerging diseases (e.g. KHV), and can be a valuable source of information to support risk analysis. They serve as building blocks of information that will be necessary for establishing disease control and management measures. For some countries, the reporting system triggered the development and establishment of surveillance systems for some of the most serious diseases occurring in the region.

Although there has been considerable progress in the implementation of the reporting system, there is still great room for advancement, particularly in developing and implementing surveillance, improving compliance, and improving the general quality of reports. Countries in which governments and policy makers have realized the trade benefits/advantages that can come with compliance to international obligations and requirements, such as international and regional disease reporting, have been quick to establish well-formulated and practical national aquatic animal health strategies with defined priorities and responsibilities for institutions and individuals. Willingness and commitment of the government, availability of technical expertise and diagnostic capabilities, and allocation of adequate resources appear

Table 3.2 List of diseases in the NACA/FAO/OIE Asia–Pacific quarterly aquatic animal disease reporting system (beginning 2004)

Diseases prevalent in the region	
OIE-listed finfish diseases	**Non OIE-listed diseases relevant in the region**
Epizootic hematopoietic necrosis	Epitheliocystis
Infectious hematopoietic necrosis	Grouper iridoviral disease
Oncorhynchus masou virus disease	Infection with koi herpes virus
Spring viraemia of carp	–
Viral hemorrhagic septicemia	–
Viral encephalopathy and retinopathy	–
Infectious pancreatic necrosis	–
Epizootic ulcerative syndrome (EUS)	–
Bacterial kidney disease	–
Red seabream iridoviral disease	–
Enteric septicemia of catfish	–
OIE-listed mollusc diseases	**Non OIE-listed diseases relevant in the region**
Infection with *Bonamia exitiosa*	Infection with *Marteilioides chungmuensis*
Infection with *Mikrocytos roughleyi*	–
Infection with *Haplosporidium nelsoni*	–
Infection with *Marteilia sydneyi*	–
Infection with *Perkinsus olseni/atlanticus*	–
OIE-listed crustacean diseases	**Non OIE-listed diseases relevant in the region**
Taura syndrome	Baculoviral midgut gland necrosis
White spot disease	Necrotising hepatopancreatitis
Yellowhead disease (YH virus, gill-associated virus)	–
Spherical baculovirosis (*Penaeus monodon*-type baculovirus)	–
Infectious hypodermal and hematopoietic necrosis	–
Spawner-isolated mortality virus disease	–
Tetrahedral baculovirosis (*Baculovirus penaei*)	–
Unknown diseases of a serious nature	
Koi mass mortality	–
Akoya oyster disease	–
Abalone viral mortality	–
Diseases presumed exotic to the region, but Listed by the OIE	
Finfish diseases	
Channel catfish virus disease	–
Infectious salmon anemia	–
Piscirickettsiosis	–
Gyrodactylosis (*Gyrodactylus salaris*)	–
White sturgeon iridoviral disease	–
Mollusc diseases	
Infection with *Bonamia ostreae*	–
Infection with *Marteilia refringens*	–
Infection with *Mikrocytos mackini*	–
Infection with *Perkinsus marinus*	–
Infection with *Candidatus Xenohaliotis californiensis*	–
Infection with *Haplosporidium costale*	–
Crustacean diseases	
Crayfish plague (*Aphanomyces astaci*)	–

to be the most important conditions for well-established disease reporting systems in some of the countries in the region.

Since 2001, the NACA/FAO/OIE QAAD list has been revised annually by the NACA Regional Advisory Group (AG) on aquatic animal health. The revisions are carried out to reflect the changes made to the OIE list of aquatic animal diseases and to include diseases of concern to the Asia–Pacific region. As a result of these revisions, the regional QAAD list, effective for reporting from the first quarter of 2004, has nine non-OIE-listed diseases relevant to the region, in addition to all of the OIE-listed diseases. As can be seen in the following section, revision of the QAAD list and inclusion of diseases of concern to the region has a positive impact on disease reporting and information sharing in the Asia–Pacific region.

In response to mass mortalities of koi and common carp in Indonesia, in 2002, "mass mortalities of koi carp" were listed under "unknown diseases of serious nature" in the FAO/NACA/OIE regional QAAD reporting list, effective for reporting from the first quarter of 2003. Since the listing of koi mass mortality in QAAD, Singapore and Thailand introduced active surveillance and quarantine programs, aimed at preventing introduction and spread of KHV.

Recognizing the importance of iridoviral disease, in terms of its potential to spread and cause economic loss, "grouper iridoviral disease" was listed in the QAAD under "any other diseases of importance," effective the first quarter of 2003. Since the listing came into effect, two countries (Hong Kong, China and Indonesia) reported positive for grouper iridoviral disease, while Singapore reported positive for mullet iridoviral disease.

Epitheliocystis, Akoya oyster disease, and the molluscan pathogen *Marteilioides chungmuensis* are of concern in the region. They were included in the QAAD list, effective the first quarter of 2003, to assist in the collection of occurrence data. Since their listing, South Korea and Japan have reported their presence.

KHV outbreaks in the region have significant trade implications for the high-value ornamental koi carp industry and the important food fish, the common carp. Active trade in ornamental fish poses a potential risk for the spread of KHV. Recognizing the significance and responding to recent confirmed KHV outbreaks in Japan, "infection with KHV" has now been added to the list of "diseases prevalent in the region" in the QAAD, effective from the first quarter of 2004.

Recognizing its potential to spread, "abalone viral mortality" has been included as an unknown disease of a serious nature in the QAAD list, effective from the first quarter of 2004. The inclusion of this disease is essential in view of the importance of mollusc aquaculture to Asia, supported by enhanced movement of their spat and adults in the region.

Information and capacity building

The NACA has conducted and/or facilitated several national and regional information and capacity building activities (Bondad-Reantaso 2001). National capacity building activities were undertaken through in-country training/workshops on various aspects of aquatic animal health management. At the regional level, several major workshops were conducted in partnership with regional and international organizations, to build consensus and promote awareness in participating governments. The FAO and NACA initiated molluscan health management in 1998, when two regional training workshops were held to build capacity in the region for molluscan disease diagnosis and management. In addition, NACA hosts the Asian Chapter of the FAO Aquatic Animal Pathogen and Quarantine Information System, an internet-based information system that supports science-based risk assessments for the movement of live aquatic animals (AAPQIS 2004).

Import risk analysis

Recognizing the increasing serious socio-economic, environmental, and possible international trade consequences arising from disease incursions related to the introduction and spread of trans-boundary pathogens/diseases through irresponsible movement of live aquatic animals, an APEC Fisheries Working Group-funded project, APEC FWG 01/2002, "Capacity and Awareness Building on IRA for Aquatic Animals," was successfully implemented by NACA during 2002–2004 in partnership with several regional and international organizations (Arthur and Bondad-Reantaso 2004).

The Project directly supported six global and regional efforts on aquatic animal health management, namely: (a) the FAO Code of Conduct for Responsible Fisheries; (b) WTO's Sanitary and Phytosanitary Agreement; (c) FAO/NACA Regional project on "Assistance for the Responsible Movement of Live Aquatic Animals in Asia"; (d) the NACA/FAO/OIE Asia–Pacific QAAD reporting system; (e) the World Bank/World Wildlife Fund [WWF]/FAO/NACA Consortium on Shrimp and the Environment; and (f) the FAO Regional Technical Cooperation Programme in the Americas on Assistance to Health Management in Shrimp Aquaculture in the Americas.

Two training workshops (1–6 April 2002 in Bangkok, Thailand; 12–17 August 2002 in Mazatlan, Mexico) brought together regulatory authorities and administrators responsible for trade of live aquatic animals, and aquatic animal health specialists to share experiences, raise awareness, build capacity, and contribute to the development of a practical manual for risk analysis to support responsible aquatic animal movements. The project provided valuable regional training and learning opportunities for APEC economies, NACA and FAO member governments, and participating regional/international organizations. The capacity to manage aquatic animal health, particularly through risk analysis, was enhanced, which could lead to improved aquatic animal health policies and practices in the region.

Important outputs include two significant publications: (a) a technical report (Arthur and Bondad-Reantaso 2004), which contains 25 technical papers covering the background for risk analysis, the risk analysis process, risk analysis and the WTO, country experiences, and national strategies on aquatic animal health and (b) a risk analysis manual (Arthur et al. 2004), which provides a simplified overview of the risk analysis process (including theoretical examples) to assist responsible individuals to formulate national policies and develop approaches to conduct risk analysis. These two publications provide further guidance to the region in the development of health management measures based on understanding and analysis of risk, a key element of the WTO-SPS Agreement and the Technical Guidelines. In addition, the publications support national efforts in import risk analyses, and contribute to the standardization of approaches by defining criteria, trade issues, and regional and international issues that will enable harmonization of import risk-assessment procedures and processes, including health certification requirements for import/export of aquatic animals across countries and across regions.

Asia regional advisory group on aquatic animal health

A regional AG on aquatic animal health was established by the Governing Council of NACA, in 2001, to accelerate the implementation of the Technical Guidelines. The AG functions as an official regional expert group to ensure that expert advice is provided to Asian governments in the implementation of the Technical Guidelines. The NACA provides institutional support, the FAO, OIE, and the identified experts provide technical guidance. The AG implements the following activities: (a) review and evaluation of regional aquatic animal disease reporting; (b) review and evaluation of implementation of the Technical Guidelines; (c) advice on identifying and designating regional aquatic animal health resources, including specialist advisers, regional reference laboratories (RRL), and resource centres; (d) revision of the Technical Guidelines (FAO/NACA 2000), the *Manual of Procedures* (FAO/NACA 2001), and the *Asia Diagnostic Guide to Aquatic Animal Diseases* (Bondad-Reantaso et al. 2001a, 2001b as required; and (e) development of procedures for dealing with aquatic animal health emergencies. Members of the AG include invited aquatic animal disease experts, the OIE, the FAO, and collaborating regional organizations. The AG meets annually, and through its meeting reports (NACA 2004), provides specialist advice to governments in the region. The first and second meetings of the AG were held in November 2002 and 2003, respectively. The NACA facilitates the implementation of the mandate of the AG and works closely with the OIE and FAO to promote the role of the region in influencing international standard setting and trade policies.

Regional resource base for aquatic animal health

Identification and establishment of the Regional Aquatic Animal Health Resource Base was one of the key recommendations of the first regional advisory group (AG-1) meeting in 2002. The resource base in aquatic animal health has been proposed at three levels: regional resource experts (RRE), regional resource centres (RRC), and RRL. The first level needed in a region is that of the RRE, to provide specialist advice to NACA in their field of expertise, assist in developing diagnostic manuals, and provide diagnostic assistance on disease emergencies in the region. The second level of resource, the RRC, is not to be specific for a single disease, but will have good experience in diagnosing and studying aquatic animal disease(s)/pathogen(s). The third level, the RRL, would be identified for diseases of regional concern not listed by the OIE, but included in the QAAD list. A cohesive networking among the RRE, RRC, and RRL in the region will provide an effective, strong, and broad network of diagnostic support that will assist in building the capacity within a region for implementation of the Technical Guidelines. The envisaged resource base within the Asia region would provide national agencies with assistance in the diagnosis of key regional diseases on the regional disease list, provide more generalized support, assist in emergency response to new disease outbreaks, and act as contact centers for advice and capacity building in close cooperation with institutions of mutual interest to improve aquatic animal health.

Response to disease emergencies

For disease emergencies within the region, NACA responds proactively. In the wake of massive mortalities of common carp and koi carp, and responding to an urgent request from the Government of Indonesia, NACA, in partnership with regional and international organizations, constituted an Emergency Disease Control Task Force, in 2002, to investigate the problem and advise the government on control measures. The Task Force provided significant insight to the problem, and recommended a series of control measures (NACA/ACIAR 2002). The Task Force findings set the stage for a follow-up project assistance from FAO through a TCP, in 2003. The NACA will continue to play an active role in the event of a disease emergency. Currently, NACA is considering how to create mechanisms that would facilitate rapid response to future disease outbreaks in the region.

Conclusion

Aquaculture has suffered significant losses due to diseases. Increasing risks are foreseen in future as aquaculture continues to expand in the region. Enabling government policies, coupled with strong resolve and commitment among stakeholders, will help in controlling diseases and contribute to development of sustainable aquaculture in the region.

Most countries face significant challenges in the practical implementation of health management strategies, specifically in the areas of diagnosis, surveillance, risk analysis, emergency preparedness, and quarantine and certification programs. Further support to national and regional initiatives is essential. The strong regional cooperation seen in the past should be continued.

The Regional Aquatic Animal Health Program of NACA will be further strengthened by supporting development and implementation of aquatic animal health strategies at different levels (production/local/national/regional) in member countries. A coordinated and cooperative approach within the region will be promoted, involving participation of stakeholders, researchers, extension and development agencies, RRCs, national governments, donor agencies, regional and international organizations, non-governmental organizations, and the private sector. New issues such as food safety and the emergence of new diseases and continued introductions of exotics to the region, will be given special attention.

The purpose of the NACA health program is to reduce risks of aquatic animal disease impacting on livelihoods of aquaculture farmers, national economies, trade, and human health. Through the ongoing and future activities in the region, the long-term expected outputs of the program are:

- development and implementation of practical national aquatic animal health strategies in the Asia–Pacific;
- widespread adoption of better aquatic animal health management practices;
- improved surveillance, reporting, and response to disease emergencies;
- harmonized diagnostic procedures and approaches to risk assessment; and
- improved regional and international cooperation in aquatic animal health.

References

AAPQIS (Aquatic Animal Pathogen and Quarantine Information System). 2004. *Food and Agriculture Organization of the United Nations*. Rome, Italy. http://www.aapqis.org.

Arthur, J.R. and M.G. Bondad-Reantaso, editors. 2004. *Capacity and Awareness Building on Import Risk Analysis (IRA) for Aquatic Animals*. Proceedings of the Workshops, 1–6 April 2002,

Bangkok, Thailand and 12–17 August 2002, Mazatlan, Mexico. Asia–Pacific Economic Cooperation Fisheries Working Group (APEC FWG) 01/2002, NACA, Bangkok, Thailand. 203 pp.

Arthur, J.R., M.G. Bondad-Reantaso, F.C. Baldock, C.J. Rodgers, and B.F. Edgerton. 2004. *Manual on Risk Analysis for the Safe Movement of Aquatic Animals (FWG/01/2002)*. APEC/DoF/NACA/FAO, NACA, Bangkok, Thailand. 59 pp.

Bondad-Reantaso, M.G. 2001. Recent Asian initiatives under the NACA regional programme on aquatic animal health management. Pages 189–205 *in* Y. Inui and E.R. Cruz-Lacierda, editors. *Disease Control in Fish and Shrimp Aquaculture in Southeast Asia–Diagnosis and Husbandry Techniques*. Proceedings of the SEAFDEC-OIE seminar workshop, Iloilo City, Philippines, 4–6 December 2001. Southeast Asian Fisheries Development Center (SEAFDEC), Iloilo, Philippines.

Bondad-Reantaso, M.G. 2004a. Trans-boundary aquatic animal diseases/pathogens. Pages 9–22 *in* J.R. Arthur and M.G. Bondad-Reantaso, editors. *Capacity and Awareness Building on Import Risk Analysis for Aquatic Animals*. Proceedings of the Workshops, Bangkok, Thailand, 1–6 April 2002, and in Mazatlan, Mexico, 12–17 August 2002. APEC FWG 01/2002, NACA, Bangkok, Thailand.

Bondad-Reantaso, M.G. 2004b. Development of national strategy on aquatic animal health management in Asia. Pages 103–108 *in* J.R. Arthur and M.G. Bondad-Reantaso, editors. *Capacity and Awareness Building on Import Risk Analysis for Aquatic Animals*. Proceedings of the Workshops, Bangkok, Thailand, 1–6 April 2002, and in Mazatlan, Mexico, 12–17 August 2002. APEC FWG 01/2002, NACA, Bangkok, Thailand.

Bondad-Reantaso, M.G., S.E. McGladdery, I. East, and R.P. Subasinghe, editors. 2001a. *Asia Diagnostic Guide to Aquatic Animal Diseases*. FAO Fisheries Technical Paper, No. 402, Suppl. 2. FAO, Rome, Italy. 236 pp.

Bondad-Reantaso, M.G., S. Kanchanakhan, and S. Chinabut. 2001b. Review of grouper diseases and health management strategies for groupers and other marine fishes. Pages 121–146 *in* M.G. Bondad-Reantaso, J. Humphrey, S. Kanchanakhan, and S. Chinabut, editors. *Development of a Regional Research Programme on Grouper Virus Transmission and Vaccine Development (APEC FWG 02/2000)*. Report of a Workshop, Bangkok, Thailand, 18–20 October 2000. Asia Pacific Economic Cooperation (APEC), Fish Health Section of the Asian Fisheries Society (FHS-AFS), Aquatic Animal Health Research Institute (AAHRI) and Network of Aquaculture Centres in Asia–Pacific (NACA), Bangkok, Thailand.

Chayaburakul, K., G. Nash, P. Pratanpipat, S. Sriurairatana, and B. Withyachumnarnkul. 2004. Multiple pathogens found in growth-retarded back tiger shrimp *Penaeus monodon* cultivated in Thailand. *Diseases of Aquatic Organisms* 60:89–96.

Cowley, J., R. McCullough, S. Kirsten, C. Lee, and P. Walker. 2002. Preliminary molecular and biological characterisation of Mourilyan virus (MoV): A new bunya-related virus of penaeid prawns. Page 103 *in Book of Abstracts*, Fifth Symposium on Diseases in Asian Aquaculture. Brisbane, Australia, 25–28 November 2002. Fish Health Section, Asian Fisheries Society, Manila, Philippines.

FAO (Food and Agriculture Organization of the United Nations). 1995. *Code of Conduct for Responsible Fisheries*. FAO, Rome, Italy. 41 pp.

FAO/NACA (Food and Agriculture Organization of the United Nations/Network of Aquaculture Centres in Asia–Pacific). 2000. *Asia Regional Technical Guidelines on Health Management for the Responsible Movement of Live Aquatic Animals and the Beijing Consensus and Implementation Strategy*. FAO Fisheries Technical Paper No. 402. FAO, Rome, Italy. 53 pp.

FAO/NACA (Food and Agriculture Organization of the United Nations/Network of Aquaculture Centres in Asia–Pacific). 2001. *Manual of Procedures for the Implementation of the Asia Regional Technical Guidelines on Health Management for the Responsible Movement of Live Aquatic Animals*. FAO Fisheries Technical Paper No. 402, Suppl. 1. FAO, Rome, Italy. 106 pp.

ISID (International Society for Infectious Diseases). 2003a. *Haliotis diversicolor supertexta (Abalone) die-off in Taiwan*. Pro-Med News, 13 March 2003, On-line version, http://www.promedmail.org. ISID, Boston, MA.

ISID (International Society for Infectious Diseases). 2003b. *Herpes virus kills 860 tons of carp*. Pro-Med-News, 4 November 2003, On-line version, http://www.promedmail.org. ISID, Boston, MA.

Israngkura, A. and S. Sae-Hae. 2002. A review of the economic impacts of aquatic animal diseases. Pages 253–286 *in* J.R. Arthur, M.J. Phillips, R.P. Subasinghe, M.B. Reantaso, and I.H. MacRae, editors. *Primary Aquatic Animal Health Care in Rural, Small-Scale, Aquaculture Development*. FAO Fisheries Technical Paper No. 406. FAO, Rome, Italy. 382 pp.

NACA (Network of Aquaculture Centres in Asia–Pacific). 2004. *Report of the Second Meeting of the Asia Regional Advisory Group on Aquatic Animal Health*. NACA, Bangkok. Thailand. 27 pp.

NACA/ACIAR (Network of Aquaculture Centres in Asia–Pacific/Australian Centre for International Agriculture Research). 2002. *Report of the Emergency Disease Control Task Force on a Serious Disease of Koi and Common Carp in Indonesia*. NACA, Bangkok. Thailand. 23 pp. On-line version, http://www.enaca.org/modules/mydownloads/viewcat.php?cid=21.

NACA/FAO (Network of Aquaculture Centres in Asia–Pacific/Food and Agriculture Organization of the United Nations). 2003. *Quarterly Aquatic Animal Disease Report (Asia and Pacific Region) 2003/2*, April–June 2003. NACA, Bangkok, Thailand. 55 pp. On-line version, http://www.enaca.org/modules/wfsection/article.php?articleid=7).

NACA/FAO (Network of Aquaculture Centres in Asia–Pacific/Food and Agriculture Organization of the United Nations). 2004. *Quarterly Aquatic Animal Disease Report (Asia and Pacific Region) 2003/4*, October to December 2003. NACA, Bangkok, Thailand. 44 pp. On-line version, http://www.enaca.org/modules/wfsection/article.php?articleid=7).

OIE (World Organisation for Animal Health). 2003. *Manual of Diagnostic Tests for Aquatic Animals*, 4th edition. OIE, Paris, France. 358 pp.

OIE (World Organisation for Animal Health). 2004. *Aquatic Animal Health Code*, 6th edition. OIE, Paris, France. On-line version, http://www.oie.int/eng/normes/fcode/A_sum.

Subasinghe, R.P., M.G. Bondad-Reantaso, and S.E. McGladdery. 2001. Aquaculture development, health and wealth. Pages 167–191 *in* R.P. Subasinghe, P. Bueno, M.J. Phillips, C. Hough, S.E. McGladdery, and J.R. Arthur, editors. *Aquaculture in the Third Millennium*. Technical Proceedings of the Conference on Aquaculture in the Third Millennium, Bangkok, Thailand, 20–25 February 2000. NACA, Bangkok, Thailand and FAO, Rome, Italy. 471 pp.

Widada, J.S., V. Richard, Z. Shi, D. Qian, and J.R. Bonami. 2004. Dot-blot hybridisation and RT-PCR detection of extra small virus (XSV) associated with white tail disease of prawn *Macrobrachium rosenbergii*. *Diseases of Aquatic Organisms* 58:83–87.

WTO (World Trade Organization). 1994. Agreement on the application of sanitary and phytosanitary measures. Pages 69–84 *in The Results of the Uruguay Round of Multilateral Trade Negotiations: The Legal Texts*. WTO, Geneva, Switzerland.

Chapter 4
Canada's Approach to Aquatic Animal Biosecurity: Experience and Evolution

Sharon E. McGladdery and Richard E. Zurbrigg

Abstract

Canada has had an eclectic experience with aquatic animal biosecurity, spanning the 1915 emergence of Malpeque disease in oysters in Prince Edward Island, development of fish health protection regulations in the 1970s to provide a health certification process for the expanding salmonid aquaculture industry, International Council for the Exploration of the Seas investigation of wild fish diseases, the 1990s infectious salmon anemia outbreaks in New Brunswick and infectious hematopoietic necrosis impacts on Atlantic salmon (*Salmo salar*) in the Pacific, and aquaculture–wild disease interaction studies, to the most recent biosecurity challenge in Canada, returning once again to the oysters of Atlantic Canada, with the emergence of MSX disease (caused by the protistan parasite, *Haplosporidium nelsoni*). The evolution of a federal approach in Canada to aquatic animal biosecurity measures is based on these experiences and changing international standards for surveillance and health certification.

Introduction

Aquatic biosecurity

Over the past 100 years, the world has seen an extraordinary globalization of human activities, linking animals, plants, and humans from around the world. Concomitant with this evolution has been the emergence of epidemic diseases, as naïve populations encounter new infectious challenges (Bixby 1992; Garrett 1995). Despite recognition of the disease risks inherent in active transfers of live animals, however, economics, emergency food production needs, and other social pressures continue to override precautionary measures (DeVoe 1992).

Sharon E. McGladdery, corresponding author. E-mail: mcgladderys@dfo-mpo.gc.ca

In some instances, environmental conditions may have spared naïve populations from exposure to pathogenic proliferation of "new" diseases, e.g., *Bonamia ostreae* suppression in European oysters (*Ostrea edulis*) in colder growing conditions (Elston 1988; Bower and Meyer 1999), *Mikrocytos mackini* suppression in *Crassostrea gigas* (Pacific oysters) in warmer growing conditions (Bower and Meyer 1999), and sea-side organism (SSO) disease of eastern oysters (*Crassostrea virginica*) in low salinity coastal waters of Atlantic Canada (M.F. Stephenson, Fisheries and Oceans Canada, unpublished data). Although such cases may be more common than previously thought, being revealed by sensitive molecular screening techniques that can detect lighter/earlier infections than previously possible (Walker and Subasinghe 2000), several other serious disease outbreaks have been related to human activities that bring pathogenic agents in contact with naïve hosts, under conditions conducive to pathogenic proliferation. These diseases are the focus of standards set by the World Organisation for Animal Health (Office International des Épizooties [OIE]), to prevent further exposure of naïve populations via aquatic animal trade activities. Several examples are given in the proceedings from the previous Biosecurity workshop, held at Honolulu in July 2001 (Lee and O'Bryen 2003).

The term "biosecurity" is well defined by other authors in this volume. For the purposes of discussion of aquatic biosecurity in the federal Canadian context, however, the term is focused on protection of naïve populations from the introduction of significant infectious diseases. This encompasses prescriptive measures for known pathogen threats as well as generic approaches for outbreaks of "new" diseases. The Canadian approach to these scenarios shares the same objectives as those of other countries faced with such challenges, i.e., accurate identification of the risk, and balance of the minimum investment required to provide acceptable risk reduction.

Effective disease prevention in the aquatic environment

In the animal world, few scenarios present more of a biosecurity challenge than those involving the open aquatic environment. Practical isolation of animals from their aquatic surroundings is limited to a small sector of the aquaculture industry. Close observation of underwater animal health requires advanced technology or investment in SCUBA diving expertise, while signs of infection are often cryptic or non-pathognomic. Open-water or flow-through aquaculture or fishing sites are subject to impacts from multiple users with widely differing socio-economic values and priorities. All of these factors are overlain by environmental influences that can affect the pathogen, as well as the host (sedentary, migratory, or farmed). Land-based farms and a longer history of knowledge about terrestrial animal diseases provide a greater number of prescriptive options for disease containment and eradication, than in aquatic settings. Shared factors, however, in the success of any disease control include effective effluent and upstream influent controls, as well as control of human activities on and among farms.

Since there can be a plethora of influences on an open-production environment, efforts must be focused on those factors that pose the highest risks. This should not ignore the lower risk vectors, but include capacity to address these as effectively as possible, albeit with less investment of resources. The Food and Agriculture Organization of the United Nations (FAO) has looked at safe trans-boundary movement of live aquatic animals using three levels of surveillance, in recognition of differing aquatic animal health infrastructure within a region (e.g., Asia). This does not reduce the protection levels to the lowest common denominator, but provides a regional network that can be used to train the people needed to build this capacity (FAO/NACA 2000, 2001; Bondad-Reantaso et al. 2001). This approach can also be applied to large countries, such as Canada, where aquatic animal health resources and expertise vary regionally.

Since options for effective disease eradication via reactive control measures are limited in open-water aquaculture production, and are virtually impossible for open-water wild populations, legislative/regulatory controls in Canada have focused on prevention. Effective proactive measures are an ongoing challenge in the light of rapid intensification and diversification of aquaculture, as well as increasing scientific knowledge about significant and new aquatic pathogens. Striking the right balance to achieve strong but flexible regulation is contingent on having a strong science basis.

The World Trade Organization (WTO) has developed the WTO Agreement on the Application of Sanitary and Phytosanitary Measures (the SPS Agreement) to which Canada and 146 other countries are signatories (WTO 2004). The science standards for disease controls are set by the World Organisation for Animal Health (OIE [formerly the Office International des Épizooties]), which has an Aquatic Animal Health Standards Commission (AAC) (the AAC [formerly the Fish Disease Commission]) to deal specifically with aquatic animal surveillance, zonation, and diagnostic standards (Bernoth this volume).

Introduction of Canada to aquatic animal health management

Malpeque disease

The first experience of a significant aquatic animal disease in Canada pre-dates modern aquatic pathology, and aquaculture, by almost 60 years. Mass mortalities of Eastern (American) oysters (*Crassostrea virginica*) occurred in Malpeque Bay, one of the major oyster-producing beds on Prince Edward Island (PEI) in 1915 (Needler and Logie 1947), but were not recognized as being due to an infectious disease, and the mortalities spread to neighboring oyster beds on PEI via transplant activities in the 1930s. At this point, the disease became known as Malpeque Bay disease, after the location where it was first recorded. Although the causative agent has not yet been conclusively determined, the disease was reported to the Royal Society of Canada by Needler and Logie (1947) with the explanation, "*. . . this account is presented because of the rarity of recorded cases of mortalities in the sea attributable to contagious disease.*" Ironically, the now internationally renowned "Malpeque oyster" derives its name from the same Bay and from the survivors of the original Malpeque disease outbreak.

Historic anecdotal evidence suggests that Malpeque disease may have been introduced via a massive transplantation of healthy oyster seeds from New England in 1913–1914 (R.E. Drinnan personal communication, September 13, 1991). This was undertaken to help restore the oyster beds in Malpeque Bay, which had shown significant stock declines due to over-fishing between 1890 and 1910. The first losses of over 99% of market size oysters in Malpeque Bay led to closure of the fishery in the Bay and movement of fishing effort to other PEI oyster beds. Between 1935 and 1937, however, the oyster stocks in Malpeque Bay had recovered to a level where they could be commercially fished again. Seed was collected and transplanted onto neighboring bays. The resultant spread of Malpeque disease virtually wiped out the remaining PEI oyster fishery. The recovered oysters from Malpeque Bay showed the first evidence of healthy carriers being responsible for the spread of an infectious agent in the marine environment; and the first Canadian aquatic biosecurity control measure was put into place. This was a complete prohibition of any oyster transfers out of PEI (Needler and Logie 1947).

The 1930s containment of oyster movements out of PEI proved successful for another 20 years, and the disease-tolerant oysters from Malpeque Bay were productive enough to replenish PEI oyster beds over that period. Effective biosecurity, however, is a double-edged sword, and human memory can rarely keep risk in perspective, especially when the supposedly risky stocks are healthy. Although the Northumberland Strait acted as an effective barrier against the spread of Malpeque from PEI across to New Brunswick (NB) for approximately 20 years, between 1952 and 1955, severe mortalities appeared in Kent County, NB, which spread north and south over a short period of time. Since Malpeque disease has an incubation period of 1 year before clinical signs appear, and mortalities occur 18–24 months post-exposure in naïve populations, it is likely that apparently healthy oysters may have been moved for up to 2 years before detection of the infection. Passive transmission via hydrographic circulation was contraindicated by the pattern of disease spread and its virulence to naïve stocks; thus, movement of infected but healthy oysters from PEI to NB was suspected (R.E. Drinnan personal communication, September 13, 1991).

At this point, an innovative approach—one that would attract strong debate in today's biosecurity arena (see Reporting and interpretation of Emergency Surveillance Results)—was implemented. It involved actively spreading PEI oysters throughout the southern Gulf of St. Lawrence (Found and Logie 1957; Drinnan 1967). The rationale was that replacement of naïve stocks with Malpeque-tolerant oysters would be the most expeditious method to accelerate recovery of the fishery from inevitable spread of the disease to neighboring NB and Nova Scotia oyster beds. This strategy worked well, and the southern Gulf of St. Lawrence now thrives on healthy, Malpeque disease-tolerant oyster populations (Fig. 4.1). Clinical signs of the disease are rare, and only naïve stocks transplanted for experimental purposes from neighboring Cape Breton waters succumb to the disease, usually within 12–18 months (McGladdery and Bower 1999; McGladdery and Stephenson 1999).

Although the gross and histopathological signs of Malpeque disease are distinctive (Fig. 4.2), the causative agent has defied conclusive identification over the past 68 years. Many organisms and etiologies have been attributed to the disease (Fraser unpublished 1939 report; Li et al. 1980), with current research indicating a possible cryptic viral or microcellular protistan etiology (McGladdery and Bower 1999). The rapid (single generation) development of tolerance in the few survivors of initial exposure to infection and the lack of a microscopically evident or culturable microbial agent have complicated the understanding of this disease. Whatever the causative agent, it is known to persist at levels infective to naïve oysters, 40 years after the last clinical outbreak (McGladdery and Stephenson 1999). Experimental transplants, however, of oysters from Cape Breton to the southern Gulf of St. Lawrence to pursue these investigations were halted in 2002 with the emergence of MSX disease (caused by *Haplosporidium nelsoni*) in oysters from inner Cape Breton waters (see Canada's reality check).

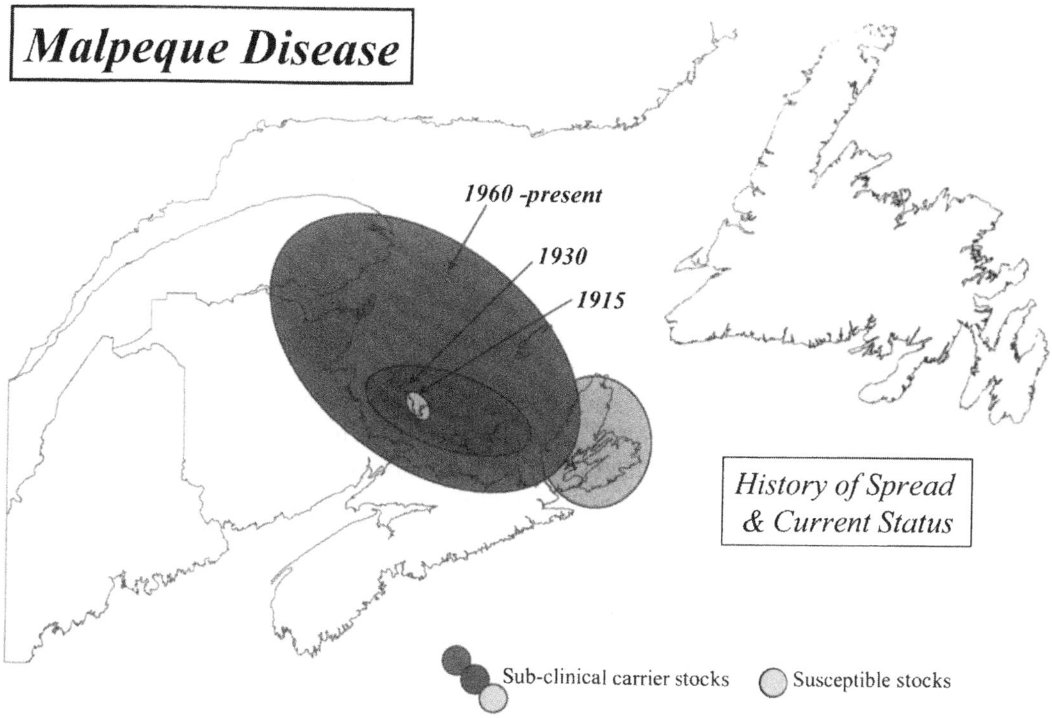

Fig. 4.1 Map of Malpeque Bay disease of Eastern oysters (*Crassostrea virginica*), its spread throughout the southern Gulf of St. Lawrence and current status.

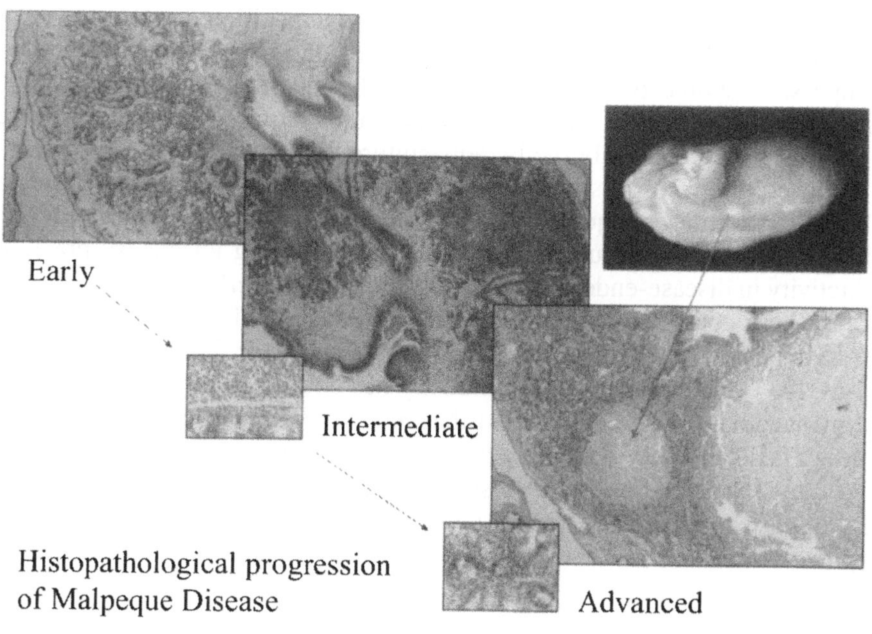

Fig. 4.2 Malpeque Bay disease histopathology and progression in *Crassostrea virginica* transplanted from Bras d'Or Lakes to the southern Gulf of St. Lawrence following 12–16 months cohabitation.

Sadly, one of the pioneers of aquatic biosecurity arising from the Malpeque oyster disease experience, Mr. Roy Drinnan, passed away in 2003, before the enigmatic cause of the disease could be determined. This was shortly after the first detection of MSX disease in the Cape Breton oysters that he and the others had so successfully protected from Malpeque disease for over 50 years.

In summary, the introduction of Canada to aquatic animal health biosecurity is founded on an etiological mystery.

Aquatic animal health management in Canada

Salmonid aquaculture

Knowledge of aquatic animal disease has grown in Canada along with the salmonid aquaculture industry since the early 1970s. Many diseases, such as bacterial kidney disease, Furunculosis, Enteric Red-Mouth, and Cold Water Vibriosis, which can be controlled today through enhanced husbandry, vaccines, and therapeutants, triggered original disease research, management, and control efforts in Canada. These diseases posed significant challenges in the 1970s and 1980s, a history well-documented in the early aquaculture pathology literature, as well as by organizations such as the International Council for the Exploration of the Sea (ICES) Working Group on Pathology and Diseases of Marine Organisms. At the same time, wild fisheries were experiencing their first recorded epidemics, and parallel discussions in the 1980s and the 1990s focused on mass mortalities in the context of fisheries management and environmental changes (Bucke et al. 1996; Wosniok et al. 2000). One example experienced by Canada was the outbreak of *Ichthyophonus hoferi* that caused mass mortalities of herring (*Clupea harengus harengus* L.) in the southern Gulf of St. Lawrence in the 1950s (Sindermann 1956). The juxtaposition of diseases in both aquaculture and wild populations has meant that the approach to health management in Canada has encompassed the objective of protection of both wild and aquaculture resources. This is a challenging balance, since the mitigative measures required to protect wild resources are, almost without exception, borne by aquaculture (Alderman 2001). Furthermore, protection of aquaculture resources from diseases endemic to surrounding wild stocks is also among the responsibilities of aquaculture. Since removal/reduction of disease levels in wild resources is impossible, aquaculture is tasked with balancing husbandry practices to ensure productivity in disease-endemic waters. Salmon (*Salmo salar* and *Oncorhynchus* spp.) producers on both coasts of Canada face this challenge, and provincially led veterinary programs have been developed to assist them in this endeavor. Through local and national associations, the Canadian aquaculture industry has addressed this challenge by developing good management practices (GMPs) that involve community as well as government input. These GMPs are now becoming established in major aquaculture producing areas of Canada (notably on the east and west coasts, for both salmonids and shellfish), with husbandry disease management, record-keeping, and health certification approaches that enhance proactive disease prevention (D. Rideout personal communication, March 2004).

Canada's fish health protection regulations

Regulatory fish health controls were not pursued until the 1970s, when live transfers of salmonids for aquaculture purposes were recognized as posing a clear risk for disease spread

(Carey 1992). In 1977, Fish Health Protection Regulations (FHPR) for Canada, promulgated under Canada's Fishery Act, were seen at the time as an effective biosecurity measure, being one of the first set of national regulations to apply to salmonid health protection (DFO 1984). Interim amendments were made to the FHPR in 1997, pending review of regulatory options for expansion to include non-salmonid species. This review process is now being influenced by frequent and significant changes in international standards, as reflected by many revisions of the International Code on Aquatic Animal Health over the past 9 years. The OIE Aquatic Code is now in its 7th edition (OIE 2004), and the Manual of Diagnostic Tests for Aquatic Animals (OIE 2003) that provides the technical guidelines to support the Code is currently undergoing a 5th revision. The rapidly evolving world of aquatic animal health knowledge poses a significant challenge to regulators who must incorporate flexibility into traditionally prescriptive legislative frameworks.

Canada's fishery (general) regulations

The Fishery (General) Regulation of Canada, under the Fisheries Act, provides a regulatory mechanism, under Section 56, to assess ecological, health, and genetic risks posed by proposed transfers of live aquatic organisms destined for release or holding in fish habitat. The provincially based, DFO Chaired, Introductions and Transfers Committees (ITCs), which recognizes that provinces have different aquaculture and wild resource protection issues, manages this risk assessment process. The Regulation resembles both the original and the revised Codes of Conduct (ICES 1984, 1988, 1995, 2003 and is the regulatory basis for Canada's National Code of Practice for the Introduction and Transfers of Aquatic Organisms (herein the National Code [DFO 2003]). This National Code was developed as a risk-assessment guideline for the ITCs in Canada. Transfer licenses issued under Section 56 of the FGA can require health reports/certification for inter-provincial movements of aquatic animals (e.g., FHPR certification for salmonids and their eggs), containment, quarantine, and reporting of abnormal mortalities to DFO authorities, as conditions of the license.

Current aquatic animal health activities

As noted in the Introduction, this chapter focuses on the federal system in Canada. The federal role of Canada is currently focused on regulatory surveillance in support of health certification and transfer license recommendations, as well as research to support risk assessments, diagnostic standards, and new pathogen identification. Research is commonly undertaken in collaboration with provincial and academic expertise. The DFO has three aquatic animal health centers, located at: the Pacific Biological Station (PBS), Nanaimo, British Columbia; the Freshwater Institute (FWI) in Winnipeg, Manitoba; and the Gulf Fisheries Centre (GFC) in Moncton, NB. The Canadian federal Aquatic Animal Health Office (AAH), located in DFO headquarters in Ottawa, Ontario, manages the activities of these centers.

The Pacific Biological Station, Nanaimo, British Columbia

The PBS is currently the sole OIE reference laboratory for Denman Island Disease of oysters (*C. gigas* and *Ostrea conchaphila* [= *lurida*], and experimentally in *C. virginica*, and *O. edulis*), with over 40 years of research experience (Quayle 1961; Bower 1988; Hervio et al. 1996; Hine et al. 2001; Joly et al. 2001). The causative agent, *M. mackini*, is a protistan with no known phylogenetic affinities (Carnegie et al. 2003). The PBS has also led research on many other diseases that have posed a health challenge to shellfish growers on the Pacific coast of Canada (e.g., nocardiosis of edible [European] oysters, *O. edulis* and *C. gigas, Perkinsus qugwadi* of Japanese scallops, *Patinopecten yessoensis,* Scallop Protistan with a "ghosty" appearance [SPG] disease of Japanese scallops [Bower et al. 1992], spotted prawn disease in Pandalids, haemic neoplasias in blue and gallo mussels [*Mytlius edulis, M. galloprovincialis*] and parasitic castrators of mussels, and geoduck abscess lesions). Information on these, and a broad list of other diseases of shellfish, is available from a web site run out of the PBS (Bower and McGladdery 2003).

Several internationally recognized pioneers of fish health and parasitology, notably, Drs. Leo Margolis, Neil Bourne, Garth Traxler, and Bob Kabata, founded the Fish Health Unit at PBS. Their research experience has provided a strong diagnostic and research foundation for fish health at PBS, with current work focusing on infectious haematopoietic necrosis in Pacific and Atlantic salmon, *Kudoa* disease in processed salmon meat, and wild-cultured salmonid sea-lice interactions. Since the British Columbia Ministry of Agriculture, Fisheries and Forestry (BCMAFF) has the regulatory authority for aquaculture management, the province is also the lead for fish farm health management. As a result, DFO and BCMAFF work closely together to ensure that surveillance activities encompass the wild and cultured data needed for health certification. In British Columbia, a strong aquatic veterinarian community that works closely with the province, further reinforces aquaculture health management.

In addition to research, the PBS Fish Health Unit is responsible for FHPR certification of salmon enhancement hatcheries in British Columbia and the Yukon. The British Columbia Fish Health Policy covers certification of commercial fish farms, licensed under provincial jurisdiction. This policy covers FHPR requirements and adopts additional measures to meet provincially set levels of health protection for salmon aquaculture. The PBS has three Local Fish Health Officers (LFHOs), who are responsible for signing FHPR certificates for the enhancement hatcheries, as well as for private growers wishing to be included in the FHPR program.

The Freshwater Institute, Winnipeg, Manitoba

The FWI is dedicated to FHPR diagnostic support for freshwater aquaculture facilities, investigative work on fish kills, and certification of fish products where required for export. The FWI Fish Health Unit also participates in the Great Lakes Fish Health Committee, and works closely with the provincial agencies responsible for fisheries and aquaculture management in Ontario, Manitoba, Saskatchewan, Alberta, Nunavut, and the Northwest Territories. This collaboration for sample collection and diagnostic support covers the huge geographic expanse of central Canada. Recent establishment of the Canadian Cooperative Wildlife Health Centre (CCWHC), centered at the University of Saskatoon Veterinary College in Saskatchewan, is also expanding the scope for enhanced collaborative diagnostic coverage of Canadian freshwater resources.

Expertise on marine mammal diseases is also located at the FWI. Although not a core component of the federal aquatic animal health surveillance and certification program, marine mammal health threats are receiving increasing attention in the biosecurity context. Researchers at FWI are working with the Canadian Food Inspection Agency (CFIA), Health Canada, the CCWHC, the Atlantic Veterinary College, and DFO marine mammal pathology expertise at the Institute Maurice Lamontagne in Québec, on health risks posed by marine mammals released from rehabilitation centers (often located far from the point of capture or release). Canada has several endangered marine mammal populations that could be at risk if exposed to animals harboring terrestrial or exotic infections that would not otherwise be encountered in the wild (Nielsen et al. 2001a, 2001b). Note that these studies are focused on diseases of the marine mammals and not on zoonoses, which are managed by Health Canada in collaboration with the CFIA and DFO.

The Gulf Fisheries Centre, Moncton, NB

The GFC is located in the "Hub" of the Maritimes, with easy access to the southern Gulf of St. Lawrence, the Bay of Fundy, and the Atlantic coast of Nova Scotia. The GFC laboratory has expertise in both fish and shellfish health. The Shellfish Health Unit provides diagnostic and research support services for Québec, NB, Prince Edward Island, Nova Scotia, and Newfoundland. It also provides health inspections and health reports that are used by the ITCs in each of these provinces to assess potential health risks posed by proposed transfers. Since October 2002, the Shellfish Health Unit has been working closely with all the Atlantic provincial agencies to help prevent the spread of MSX disease from Cape Breton waters to uninfected oyster stocks in the southern Gulf of St. Lawrence (see Canada's reality check). Other ongoing works include analysis of the cause and epidemiology of Malpeque disease (see Malpeque disease), examination of mass mortalities of soft-shell clams (*Mya arenaria*) associated with hemic neoplasia, and risk assessment for transfers of mussels infected by parasitic digenean castrators (e.g., *Prosorhynchus squamatous*).

The Fish Health Unit is responsible for FHPR certification of aquaculture facilities throughout Atlantic Canada, including Newfoundland and Quebec. Several non-DFO laboratories also provide this service through Fish Health Officials (FHOs) designated to undertake FHPR inspections on behalf of DFO. The GFC has two LFHOs responsible for signing FHPR certificates. The Fish Health Unit is also responsible for investigating wild fish kills, dealing with new disease outbreaks, and health-screening exotic species brought into Canada for research purposes. Both the Shellfish and Fish Health Units are responsible for inspecting quarantine or containment facilities used for research purposes of live-holding of species or stocks that have inadequate or high-risk health histories.

An important component of both finfish and shellfish diagnostics is field validation of the growing number of molecular tests that are emerging for known infectious agents. Most are aimed at early and rapid identification of infections that would not be detected using more traditional screening techniques. As the scope of their use increases (geographically and for a wider range of species), sensitivity and specificity analyses need to undergo ongoing refinement (Walker and Subasinghe 2000). The management implications of positive results that suggest the presence of infection, but which are non-repeatable or lack visual confirmation of the infectious agent, are significant. Both the PBS and GFC aquatic animal health groups are working with OIE and provincial reference laboratories to ensure that quality assurance/quality control standards for polymerase chain reaction (PCR) are reliable (Chapter 1.1.3. in OIE 2003).

DFO Headquarters—National capital region, Ottawa, Ontario

In 2004, the National Registry of Fish Diseases, at DFO Headquarters, was renamed the National Registry of Aquatic Animal Health (NRAAH). It is one component of the AAH. These changes reflect expansion of federal aquatic animal health responsibilities beyond management of the FHPR. The NRAAH is the archive center for FHPR health reports, certificates and related transfer and trade documentation. The NRAAH is also responsible for an advance rulings process that deals with salmonid health certification, for cases that do not meet FHPR requirements. The NRAAH also posts information on the DFO Science web-site on common certification and regulatory questions. The NRAAH is also the coordination center for ensuring that non-federal FHOs and LFHOs are kept informed of updates to the FHPR Manual of Compliance, and is the application point for people wishing to become designated FHOs or LFHOs. The NRAAH is currently revising the FHPR Manual of Compliance, in preparation for the upcoming regulatory amendments.

Other components of the AAH specialize in the regulatory amendment process, international trade certification issues (in collaboration with CFIA and International Trade Canada), federal and provincial government health management coordination, health risk analysis support for the National Code, and industry liaison for disease emergencies of national concern.

With respect to International Trade and aquatic animal health, DFO is the Competent Authority (Chapter 1.4.3. in OIE 2004) in Canada for aquatic animal health. The AAH is responsible for providing regular reports to the Chief Veterinary Officer (CVO) for Canada, located within the CFIA on OIE-related aquatic animal health matters. In addition, AAH is responsible for reviewing and providing scientific comment on proposed amendments to the OIE Aquatic Code and Manual, through the office of the CVO. The AAH is also the authority for aquatic animal health certification of product destined for import by countries or regions requiring such certification (e.g., Europe, as described by Alderman 2002).

The AAH is the management center for the web-based NRAAH database, designed to facilitate entry of presence/absence data from laboratories participating in the surveillance program for zonation of diseases of national concern. This is a layered database with data entered using a Geographic Positioning System (GPS latitude-longitude). The prototype is being tested using data gathered from DFO laboratories, covering diagnostic analyses over the last 3–5 years using standardized procedures. This is used as a primary aid to zonation for major diseases of national concern. Client details are not entered, but retained by the diagnostic laboratory to ensure rapid contact in case of a query or disease emergency. The web-based design is intended to facilitate future participation by non-federal laboratories wishing to contribute data to support mapping of diseases of national concern.

Adapting to national and international change

National changes impacting Canada's aquatic animal health program

The aquaculture sector in Canada has evolved significantly over the past 30–40 years, expanding from put-and-take rainbow trout (*Oncorhynchus mykiss*) operations to small-scale Atlantic and Pacific salmon (*Oncorhynchus* spp., *Salmo salar*) farms to full-scale, open-water and land-based production facilities. Many family-owned seed collection and relay shellfish producers of the 1960s have developed into vertically integrated international suppliers of mussels (*Mytilus edulis*), clams (*Mya arenaria, Mercenaria mercenaria, Protothaca staminea, and Tapes philippinarum*), and oysters (*Crassostrea virginica, C. gigas,* and *O. edulis*). Scallop (*Placopecten magellanicus* and *Patinopecten yessoensis*) production is not far behind in development on both coasts, and there is growing interest in northern (Pinto) abalone (*Haliotis kamtschatkana*), geoduck (*Panope abrupta*), and sea-urchin (*Strongylocentrotus droebachiensis*) culture. This diversification is a welcome evolution away from vulnerable monoculture systems, but presents a challenge in differentiating between relatively benign infections and those that threaten naïve stock. Baseline health profiles are rarely known before a new species is developed for aquaculture production. Local resources have been used to build hatchery broodstock and juvenile production for some species under culture assessment, e.g., shortnose sturgeon (*Acipenser brevirostrum*), Atlantic sturgeon (*A. oxyrhynchus*), Atlantic halibut (*Hippoglossus hippoglossus*), winter flounder (*Pleuronectes americanus*), and Atlantic haddock (*Melanogrammus aeglefinus*), and cod (*Gadus morhua*) (Litvak 1999; Martin-Robichaud 2003). Where local stocks have been unavailable or non-native species are of interest, Canada has also used quarantine to hold broodstock and to produce an F1 generation for health assessment. All (100%) of the broodstock are examined for infectious agents or signs of disease, along with a sample of the F1, when large enough to be examined. Once health inspections are complete, with no sign of infections of concern, the F1 can be released. Several introductions and transfers into and within Canada have been successfully undertaken using this ICES Code of Practice approach (Carey 1992).

Proximity exposure of the broodstock to native species was added for two introductions of bay scallops (*Argopecten irradians*), one into PEI in 1990 (Whyte et al. 1993, 1994) and another into Nova Scotia in 1990 (McGladdery et al. 1993). The proximity exposure was aimed at assessing risks to local stocks of any "new" or unidentified infectious agent that might be detected during the quarantine period. A rickettsial-like agent found during an earlier introduction of bay scallops (1983) posed a significant challenge for risk assessment. The same types of organisms are common in all molluscs, but differentiation of species or strains was difficult (predating recent advances made in molecular identification technology). After being held through four generations in quarantine, and with a decrease in infection recorded over that period, approval was given to undertake open-water, grow-out testing. Eight years later, two additional infections were detected in the bay scallops that were traced back to the original broodstock, via records of the same agents in bay scallops from Connecticut, the source of the original introduction (Karlsson 1991).

Although a costly investment, addition of local species to the quarantine containment provides enhanced confidence that any unknown pathogens found, or those that may escape detection using routine surveillance techniques, do not pose a significant health threat to local species. Use of ambient holding conditions and/or stress testing (e.g., by heat-shock) has also been used to assess the risk of cross-species transmission and pathogenicity of any unknown or undetected infectious agents (Whyte et al. 1994).

International changes impacting Canada's aquatic animal health program

The Agreement on the Application of Sanitary and Phytosanitary Measures (SPS Agreement) of the WTO provides a comprehensive set of guidelines that trade partners can use to establish harmonized disease surveillance and health certification standards (WTO 2004). The SPS Agreement consists of 14 Articles with three Annexes encompassing Definitions; Transparency of Regulations; and Control, Inspection, and Approval Procedures. Canada signed the SPS Agreement in 1995, joining 146 other countries that are now signatories. The scientific standard setting body for animal health surveillance and certification is the OIE. The AAC of the OIE review and publish the requirements for safe trade in aquatic animals and their products in the OIE Aquatic Animal Health Code (OIE Aquatic Code) as online and paper copies (OIE 2004), and the Manual of Diagnostic Tests for Aquatic Animals (OIE Manual), also online and paper copies (OIE 2003).

Recent changes in the OIE Aquatic Code and Manual have significantly expanded the lists of potentially susceptible species or species-groups. This is based on field observations, as well as *in vitro per os* and inoculation laboratory challenge experiments. These changes have increased the pressure on countries with host populations that are positive for a reportable disease, to provide evidence on whether or not sympatric species (up to Class) present a risk of pathogen transmission.

The revisions to the national aquatic animal health program (NAAHP) for Canada include risk analysis investigation, where warranted by export and/or aquaculture development interests, to assess certification requirements for sympatric species in endemic areas. Although protocols for assessing risk of disease transmission via sub-clinical infections in abnormal hosts have yet to be defined, several countries and regions have introduced legislation that is not host species-specific. The potential impact on polyculture and other aquatic resource users in areas positive for an OIE-listed disease, therefore, requires focused risk assessment. Since detection and identification of known pathogens in abnormal hosts that show no clinical sign of infection is a challenge, Canada is currently assessing the efficacy of PCR technology as a primary screening tool. The pitfalls inherent in molecular test screening have been well described (Walker and Subasinghe 2000), and are being taken into account for interpretation of results. Canada's experience with this is described further under "Canada's reality check: MSX, a case study."

Canada's national aquatic animal health partnership

Several provinces have developed comprehensive fish health programs, based on experience with recurrent and significant infectious diseases, principally in salmonid aquaculture. In developing these programs, the provinces highlighted the need for coordination of federal and provincial disease management efforts to optimize use of Canadian aquatic animal health expertise and resources. In 1999, the Canadian Council of Fisheries and Aquaculture Ministers (CCFAM—federal and provincial Ministers) tasked DFO with leading development of a federal-provincial-industry NAAHP. Discussions were initiated in April 2000, with the Canadian Aquaculture Industry Alliance representing all aquaculture sectors (shellfish and freshwater, anadromous, and marine finfish). Veterinary input was provided through provincial veterinarians, Canadian veterinary colleges, and the Canadian Veterinary Medical Association.

Over the last 4 years, the key components required for a comprehensive program have been defined, along with federal, provincial, and industry roles and responsibilities (Fig. 4.3). Industry plays the lead role for management of production (husbandry-related) diseases; the provinces lead on management of endemic diseases; and the federal government is

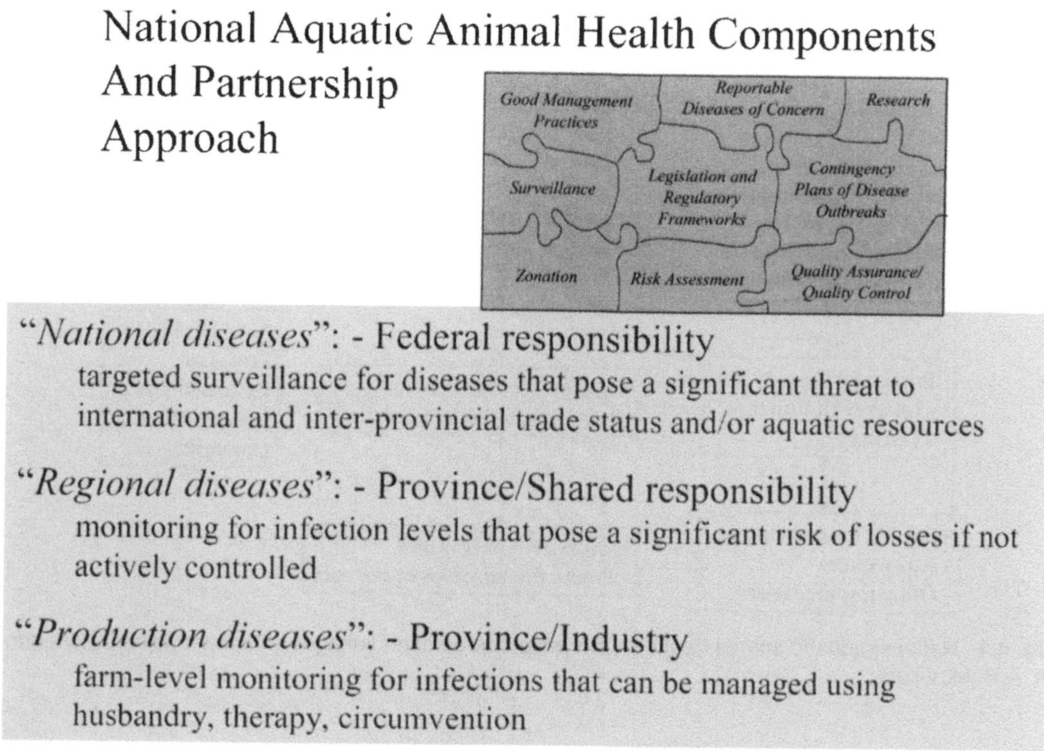

Fig. 4.3 Proposed Canadian National Aquatic Animal Health Partnership (NAAHP) components and disease management responsibilities (Jigsaw accredited to I.M. Price).

responsible for diseases that meet OIE listing criteria and are exotic to all or parts of Canada. The federal role focuses on aquatic animal health certification for the purposes of trade as well as protection of vulnerable resources.

Compliance within any disease management program is a universal challenge, and the NAAHP for Canada is no different. The range of environments, species, and resource users poses a significant challenge. Industry, as mentioned above, under salmonid aquaculture, is developing GMPs encompassing health management (transfer records, disease reporting, treatment records, etc.). These are either self-policing or required by provincial leases, subject to lease withdrawal for non-compliance. This is seen as a strong first line of defense against high disease risk activities. Federal regulatory and surveillance activities will focus on demonstrating freedom from diseases of concern through scientifically sound surveillance programs (OIE 2003; FAO 2004) supported by coordinated contingency plans. The overall program is schematically represented in Figure 4.4.

Canada's reality check: MSX, a case study

The model contingency plan

In September 2002, a model contingency plan was presented for an OIE-listed disease that would be a significant threat to a commercially significant species in Canada (S.E.

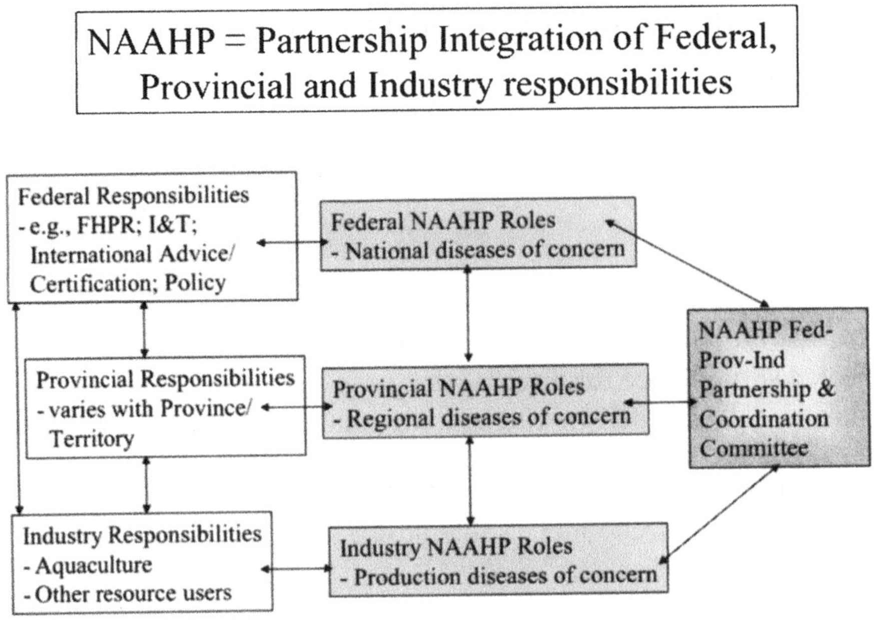

Fig. 4.4 National aquatic animal health partnership coordination linkages (original outline credited to Dr. A.H. McVicar).

McGladdery and W.S. Warrell, personal communication, September 2002). The model was aimed at defining roles, responsibilities, and resource requirements to address a disease emergency in the context of the development of the NAAHP. The model used was MSX disease of eastern oysters (*C. virginica*) caused by the parasite *Haplosporidium nelsoni*. The choice of MSX as a "worst case scenario" was because detection of sub-clinical infections is difficult using routine histopathology screening techniques, the mechanism(s) of transmission are unknown, and the parasite shows no predilection for aquaculture or wild oysters, making isolation of affected stocks in open-water "problematic." Furthermore, in the Canadian context, oyster production spans federal and provincial authorities, with stakeholders encompassing First Nations' traditional food fisheries, commercial fisheries interests, provincially licensed aquaculture lease-holders, CFIA-registered processing plants, and brokerage operations, as well as live marketers using roadside trucks, local stores, and commercial distribution centers.

At the same time, oyster samples from St. Patrick's Channel, an entry channel to Bras d'Or Lakes in central Cape Breton, Nova Scotia (Fig. 4.5), had been submitted to the DFO Shellfish Health Unit in Moncton, due to reports of increasing levels of mortality during 2002. Examination of the samples revealed plasmodial-like inclusions, hitherto unseen in Canadian oyster samples. The level of infection, along with extensive hemocyte infiltration, indicated that this was the likely cause of the mortalities. Histopathology samples were immediately sent to the PBS, and the Oxford Maryland Cooperative Laboratory. Histopathology and tissue samples preserved for molecular analysis were sent to the OIE reference laboratory at the Virginia Institute of Marine Sciences (VIMS), Williamsburg, Virginia.

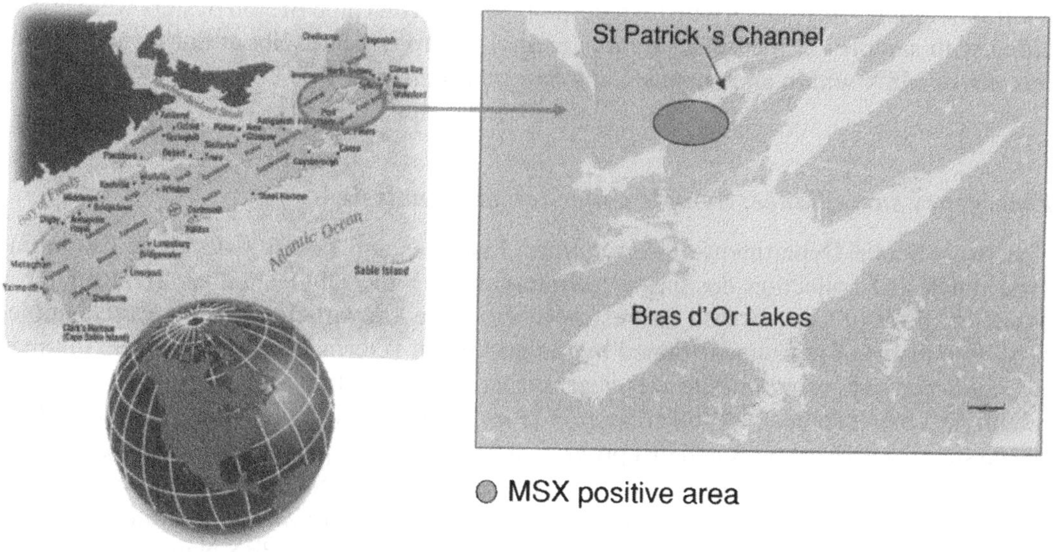

Fig. 4.5 St. Patrick's Channel, Cape Breton, where MSX was first detected in eastern oysters (*Crassostrea virginica*) in October 2002 (globe and Nova Scotia map obtained from www.gov.ns.ca/nsmap.htm).

A working contingency plan

The model contingency plan was converted to a working contingency plan prior to official confirmation of the diagnosis. Principal DFO and provincial personnel were alerted and tasked with contacting the directly affected stakeholders, and preparing information for the public and for media communications. Aquaculture industry divers who were inspecting the extent of the mortalities collected additional samples. These were the last Cape Breton oyster samples collected without official government (federal or provincial) oversight.

The OIE reference laboratory at VIMS confirmed MSX on 18 October 2002, the CVO for Canada was notified, and a report was sent to the OIE headquarters in Paris. The report provided information on the known geographic extent of infection, the mortality levels being reported, the contingency plan, and the surveillance plans to delineate the exact geographic extent of the distribution of MSX in Canadian eastern oyster stocks (Stephenson et al. 2003).

Meetings were held with Cape Breton oyster growers, First Nations, provincial and federal fisheries, and seafood authorities. They were presented with an overview of what was known about MSX, and consulted on the possible scenarios, for introduction of the disease along with immediate control options. The possibility for a historic presence of the infection in Bras d'Or Lakes was also discussed. The reported high (80–90%) mortalities and stages of infection found, however, appeared to be more indicative of a point source outbreak. Using the information on hand, surveillance was aimed at determining how far the disease could have spread outward from the known infection area.

Surveillance strategies focused on current and recent oyster transfers within and out of Cape Breton waters. Trace backs showed links to the southern Gulf of St. Lawrence and Prince Edward Island, over the previous 2 years, for live-holding, processing, and depuration relay. Neighboring provinces were alerted and included in surveillance collections. In addition, samples from areas with no record of contact with Cape Breton oysters were tested, along with samples of mussels, (*Mytilus edulis*) due to concerns about non-oyster-related transfer of MSX within and outside Cape Breton waters.

Emergency surveillance: Sample collection and analysis

The Nova Scotia Department of Agriculture, Fisheries and Forestry developed sampling procedures and collection design in consultation with the DFO Shellfish Health Unit at Moncton. Sites in Cape Breton farthest away from the known affected sites were sampled first. Two teams of personnel, trained by the provincial veterinarian, visited a maximum of two sites per day, using on-site wet gear, boats, and harvesting equipment. All materials transferred between sites by the collection team, including vehicles, were disinfected between sites. New Brunswick and PEI provincial fisheries and aquaculture authorities assisted with collections from their provinces. These collections extended into winter months, despite the challenges of remote winter travel and sampling at sub-zero temperatures through ice. Shellfish pathologists at the DFO laboratory in Moncton and PBS Nanaimo examined the samples. Sample receipt, processing, histopathology screening, data recording, and PCR sub-sample analyses were undertaken in accordance with detailed guidelines, prepared in advance by the DFO Shellfish Health Unit. Equipment was standardized to ensure that effort and results between different inspectors and analysts were consistent. This included microscope objective magnifications, the number of runs through automatic staining machines for optimum counter-stain contrast, and the equipment used for DNA extraction from tissue homogenates for PCR and for *in situ* hybridization analyses.

Due to winter temperatures being associated with lighter levels of infection in oysters in endemic waters along the eastern United States, confidence in negative results from routine microscope examinations was low, especially those collected from oysters close to known positive sites, or with direct links to affected sites. Tissue samples from all oysters collected for the initial emergency surveillance were preserved for PCR using sterile technique, to prevent cross-specimen contamination prior to collection of tissues destined for both light microscopy and electron microscopy.

Histopathology samples were examined using a protocol that covered the greatest geographic range possible, as quickly as possible, for heavy/conclusive infections. Thirty oysters, from each sample of 60, were examined at low and medium microscope magnification, considered sufficient to detect heavy infections. Once all samples had been screened at this level, all negative samples were re-examined at high-dry magnification for light infections that could have been missed at the lower microscope magnifications. Another pathologist made a third examination of any sub-clinical or inconclusive infections, for confirmation purposes. Some inconclusive samples were also sent to the OIE reference laboratory and to Dr. Susan Ford of the Haskin Shellfish Research Laboratory at Rutgers University, USA.

The remaining 30 oysters, from samples that were negative after the low- and high-power sweep, were then examined to further check for absence of MSX. Lastly, sub-samples of tissues preserved in 90% ethanol from negative oysters, along with all oysters showing inconclusive plasmodia-like tissue inclusions, were tested using the MSX-specific PCR probes developed by the OIE reference laboratory.

Throughout each analysis stage, a central logbook tracked sample progression through the examination protocols. Positive infections indicated a positive sample, but further analysis for percentage of infection and intensity was deferred until all samples had been examined.

Reporting and interpretation of emergency surveillance results

The conclusive results from the initial emergency surveillance were obtained in November 2002 and released according to a media communications plan. The results showed two apparent levels of MSX infection. One was the classic MSX infection with plasmodia proliferation throughout the connective tissues and digestive tubules, some of which also showed spore development. These were found exclusively in oysters that had direct contact with the point source in St. Patrick's Channel, Cape Breton. A second type of infection, showing isolated plasmodia with no sign of proliferation or hemocyte infiltration response, was also detected and reported as inconclusive. Results from MSX primer PCR analysis of these infections were all negative. Since this was also the case for some specimens with lighter MSX infections, the possibility of false negatives as well as false positives needed further analyses.

Tests performed using the PCR primer for SSO, an oyster disease caused by *Haplosporidium costale* and a close relative of the MSX organism, confirmed the presence of the SSO parasite in oysters from Prince Edward Island and the north shore of Cape Breton outside Bras d'Or Lakes. These infections were all light (1–3 plasmodia per tissue section) (Fig. 4.6), and had no obvious links to the MSX outbreak in Cape Breton. Since SSO was

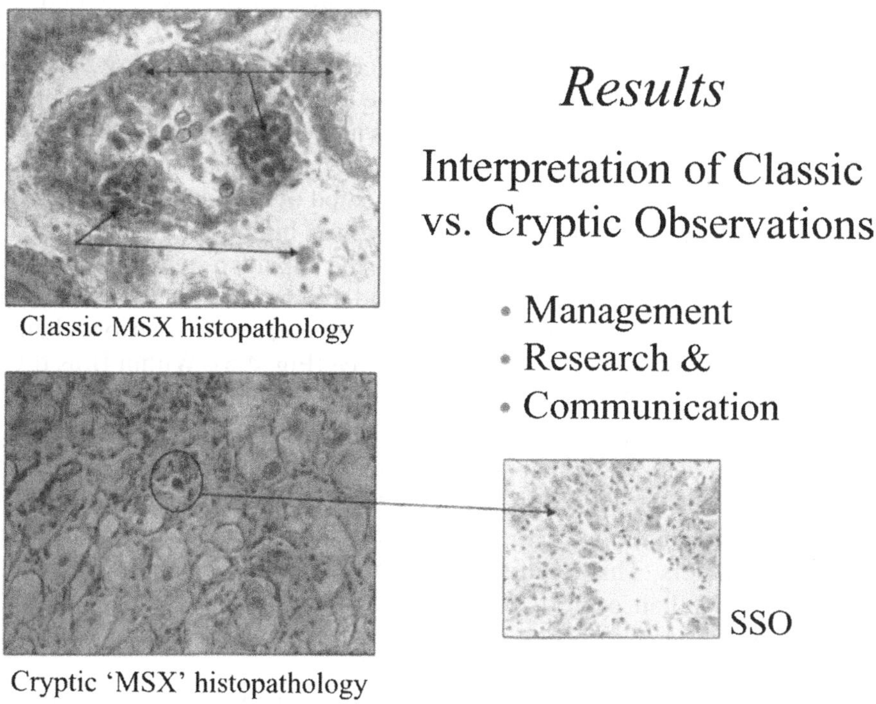

Fig. 4.6 MSX and SSO infections on Atlantic populations of eastern oysters (*Crassostrea virginica*).

listed by the OIE as one of a number of "other significant diseases" for molluscs in 2002, this was also reported to the OIE as a new finding for Canada. This was given the caveat that none of the infections were associated with evidence of disease.

Additional samples were collected over winter from wild and cultured oyster beds in Cape Breton, Nova Scotia, southwest Nova Scotia, the Bay of Fundy, and southern Gulf of St. Lawrence, NB, Prince Edward Island, and the Magdalen Islands, Québec. The results from all analyses, plus those conducted in early spring 2003, showed no change in the geographic distribution of MSX, but added more areas with sub-clinical SSO infections.

Control options and considerations

As soon as MSX was suspected, senior management were alerted that all movement of oysters out of Cape Breton should be stopped. When the disease was confirmed, the only oyster harvesting activities were those off aquaculture leases and by First Nations for their Food Fishery. The commercial fishery was closed for conservation purposes. The DFO closed the fishery and worked with the province of Nova Scotia and the oyster growers, on protocols that would permit harvesting of product but prevent spread of MSX to neighboring waters with that product. A license to harvest was issued to lease-holders who attested to washing the product on site, and had signed the agreement from a registered Cape Breton processing plant that the oysters would be subject to direct packaging (no further washing or refreshing) and distributed to markets west of Québec city. These "Harvest Protocols" were reviewed and modified, as more information became available about the distribution of MSX.

When it was determined that MSX had an apparently limited distribution within Bras d'Or Lakes, the feasibility of eradication of the disease agent was considered. A potential window of opportunity existed for oyster depopulation at affected sites in early May 2003, following ice-out and before temperatures and salinities rose to levels conducive to MSX proliferation (>10°C). Such an eradication attempt, however, was judged unrealistic, given that all oysters (spat to adults) from affected areas would need to be removed, that the intermediate host or reservoir of infection was unknown, and that the method of introduction of MSX into Bras d'Or Lakes was unknown. The potential for failure was high due to unharvested oysters, unknown reservoirs of infection, and re-exposure to the unknown source of infection. Thus, an MSX-positive zone had to be first defined around the known infected sites.

Bras d'Or Lakes are almost completely enclosed by land, with a narrow channel at the north exiting to the mouth of the Gulf of St. Lawrence (Fig. 4.5). Within Bras d'Or Lakes, isolation of affected and unaffected stocks was deemed impractical, due to the wide diversity of commercial and recreational water users. Thus, the whole system, including both positive and negative oyster stocks, was zoned positive with the objective of disease containment.

Control options based on this MSX-positive zone designation were developed. First, all ITCs were notified of the need to refuse transfer licenses for oyster movement out of Bras d'Or Lake waters. This reinforced controls already in place through the Harvest Protocols. Federal surveillance efforts concentrated on a designated buffer zone surrounding Cape Breton, to ensure early detection of any emergence of MSX outside Bras d'Or Lakes (Fig. 4.7).

Consideration was given to mass transplantation of infected stocks around Bras d'Or Lakes, for the same reasons applied to the management of Malpeque disease in the 1950s

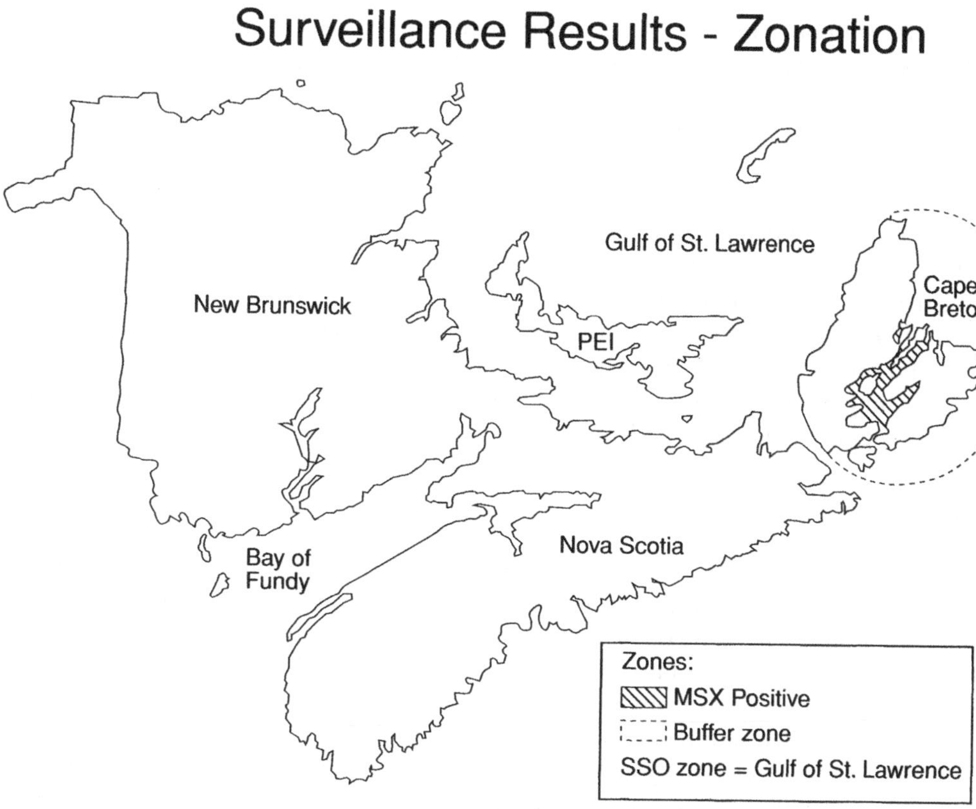

Fig. 4.7 Zonation status for MSX in Atlantic Canadian waters, July 2004.

(see Malpeque disease), to accelerate spread of the disease and depopulate remaining naïve stocks. With no concrete evidence, however, of tolerance in surviving oysters in Cape Breton, and over 40 years of selective breeding for resistance to MSX in the US (confounded by dual infection by another parasite, *Perkinsus marinus*) only now beginning to show signs of success (Ragone-Calvo et al. 2003), this control option was considered to be premature.

There also remained hope that the particularly severe winter of 2002–2003 would take a natural toll on MSX. But this proved not to be the case when the disease re-emerged in oysters from Bras d'Or Lakes in the early summer of 2003.

With respect to SSO, surveillance results showed sub-clinical infections sporadically distributed around the Atlantic provinces. Histology-based prevalence of infection in positive samples was $<5\%$, and intensity of infection <3 plasmodia/tissue section. A single coinfection with MSX was found in Cape Breton. Since SSO showed no evident pathogenic effect on infected oysters, along with an apparently broad distribution, no specific measures were introduced to control this infection. A Haplosporidian reported from a single mussel from PEI in 2002 showed no molecular affinity to either MSX or SSO (Stephenson and McGladdery 2002).

The most challenging control debate centered on whether or not transfer restrictions should be applied to other species in the MSX-positive zone (see discussion under International changes impacting Canada's aquatic animal health program). Transfers of scallops from infectious salmon anemia (ISA)-endemic areas and mussels from Malpeque-endemic areas have been subject to similar debate. The ISA screening of scallops used sensitive salmonid cell-lines. Malpeque disease risks from mussels used oyster "canary" sentinels. Neither showed any evidence of being carriers or vectors of the infectious agent of concern.

With respect to MSX risk, however, mussel transfers were prohibited pending PCR analysis of samples collected from near the most heavily MSX-positive oyster beds in late 2002. This exercise was repeated in the summer of 2003. Neither these nor the samples examined from other locations in Cape Breton showed any evidence of the presence of *H. nelsoni* or *H. costale.* Thus, no restrictions on movements of other molluscs out of the MSX-affected zone were made. Such transfers were subject to normal conditions of transfer, including washing on site to reduce the risk of transfer of fouling organisms (such as juvenile oysters) that might transmit the MSX parasite.

Current status

As noted in the section, "Reporting and interpretation of emergency surveillance results," the winter of 2002–2003 was the hardest salt-water freeze-over experienced in Atlantic Canada, for a decade. The spring thawing of the deep ice and snow cover reduced the salinities within the lakes to <15 ppt, until late into May–June in many bays. Heavy infections, however, were detected again in oysters from St. Patrick's Channel and other sites within Bras d'Or Lakes, by June 2003. These infections have persisted until 2004.

No MSX has been detected in oysters sampled outside Bras d'Or Lakes waters. Thus, the remaining oyster-producing areas in Atlantic Canada are considered negative at the time of writing. All mortalities from these areas are examined for both MSX and SSO.

The controls in place continue to require lease-holders to harvest their oysters under stringent guidelines, although options have now been expanded to permit processing outside Cape Breton, within a federally registered processing plant with effluent treatment controls. Marketing for direct human consumption is now permitted anywhere, with labeling "for direct human consumption" to reduce the risk of re-soaking.

Although these controls appear to have been effective thus far, success in preventing the spread is limited at best, and vulnerable to ignorance or deliberate circumvention. Imposing restrictions on one sector of an industry with the significant economic impacts this incurs, while neighbors conduct business as usual, requires strong risk communication to avoid "mutiny" and non-compliance.

Conclusions

Canada's aquatic animal biosecurity experience does not differ significantly from that of other countries. On the other hand, its history of disease unknowns, geographic expanse and seasonal compression of productivity, multi-user interests, and shared borders with the United States distinguishes the Canadian experience from that of many other countries and regions.

This chapter emphasizes mollusc examples. This is deliberate, in light of well-documented finfish examples covered by Canada and other countries elsewhere in this volume. The unknown issues, however, that haunt molluscan health protection technically, epidemiologically, and with respect to multi-user stakeholder interests, apply equally to domestication of future new species (finfish, molluscs, crustaceans, echinoderms, etc.).

Acknowledgments

A century of review comes with a century of acknowledgments covered, albeit insufficiently, via references and comments in the chapter. The authors express sincere thanks to the reviewers of this chapter manuscript, and acknowledge that Canada's biosecurity programs could have encompassed many more areas—certainly the Great Lakes and other freshwater or marine mammal biosecurity questions were seriously "short-changed." We hope to acknowledge these better, via future biosecurity discussions and research.

References

Alderman, D.J. 2001. Control of the spread of pathogens—The regulatory approach, its history and present status. Pages 215–231 *in* C.-S. Lee and P.J. O'Bryen, editors. *Biosecurity in Aquaculture Production Systems: Exclusion of Pathogens and Other Undesirables*. The World Aquaculture Society, Baton Rouge, LA.

Alderman, D.J. 2002. Trends in therapy and prophylaxis 1991–2001. *Bulletin of the European Association of Fish Pathologists* 22:117–125.

Bixby, D.E. 1992. Species introductions and transfers in agriculture. Pages 5–7 *in* R. DeVoe, editor. *Introductions and Transfers of Marine Species: Achieving a Balance Between Economic Development and Resource Protection*. Proceedings of the Conference and Workshop, Hilton Head Island, SC, October 30–November 2, 1991. South Carolina Sea Grant Consortium, Charleston, SC.

Bondad-Reantaso, M.G., S.E. McGladdery, I. East, and R.P. Subasinghe. 2001. *Asia Diagnostic Guide to Aquatic Animal Diseases*. FAO Fisheries Technical Paper No. 402/2. FAO and NACA (Food and Agriculture Organization of the United Nations/Network of Aquaculture Centres in Asia–Pacific), Fisheries and Agriculture Organization, Rome, Italy. 237 pp. On-line version, www.enaca.org/NACA-Publications/ADG-complete.pdf.

Bower, S.M. 1988. Circumvention of mortalities caused by Denman Island Oyster disease during mariculture of Pacific Oysters. *American Fisheries Society Special Publication* 18:246–248.

Bower, S.M. and S.E. McGladdery. 2003. *Synopsis of Infectious Diseases and Parasites of Commercially Exploited Shellfish: Introduction*. Fisheries and Oceans Canada-Pacific Region. On-line version, http://www-sci.pac.dfo-mpo.gc.ca/shelldis/title_e.htm.

Bower, S.M. and G.R. Meyer. 1999. Effect of cold water on limiting or exacerbating some oyster diseases (abstract). *Journal of Shellfish Research* 18(1):296.

Bower, S.M., J. Blackbourn, G.R. Meyer, and D.J.H. Nishimura. 1992.Diseases of cultured Japanese scallops (*Patinopecten yessoensis*) in British Columbia, Canada. *Aquaculture* 107:201–210.

Bucke, D., D. Vethaak, T. Lang, and S. Mellergaard. 1996. *Common Diseases and Parasites of Fish in the North Atlantic: Training Guide for Identification*. ICES Techniques in Marine Environmental Science, No. 19. International Council for the Exploration of the Seas (ICES), Copenhagen, Denmark. 27 pp.

Carey, T.G. 1992. Federal and provincial policies for marine species introductions and transfers in Atlantic Canada. Pages 43–46 *in* R. DeVoe, editor. *Introductions and Transfers of Marine Species: Achieving a Balance Between Economic Development and Resource Protection*. Proceedings of the Conference and Workshop, Hilton Head Island, SC, October 30–November 2, 1991. South Carolina Sea Grant Consortium, Charleston, SC.

Carnegie, R.B., G.R. Meyer, J. Blackbourn, N. Cochennec-Laureau, F.C.J. Berthe, and S.M. Bower. 2003. Molecular detection of the oyster parasite *Mikrocytos mackini* and a preliminary phylogenetic analysis. *Diseases of Aquatic Organisms* 54:219–227.

DeVoe, R.M., editor. 1992. *Introductions and Transfers of Marine Species: Achieving a Balance Between Economic Development and Resource Protection*. Proceedings of the Conference and Workshop, Hilton Head Island, SC, October 30–November 2, 1991. South Carolina Sea Grant Consortium, Charleston, SC. 198 pp.

DFO (Fisheries and Oceans Canada). 1984. *Fish Health Protection Regulations Manual of Compliance*. Miscellaneous Special Publications #31 (revised). Fisheries and Oceans Canada, Ottawa, Ontario, Canada. 42 pp.

DFO (Fisheries and Oceans Canada). 2003. *National Code on Introductions and Transfers of Aquatic Organisms*. Fisheries and Oceans Canada, Ottawa, Ontario, Canada. On-line version, www.dfo-mpo.gc.ca/science/aquaculture/code/Code2003_e.pdf.

Drinnan, R.E. 1967. Rehabilitation of disease-depleted oyster populations in Eastern Canada by large-scale transplants. *International Council for the Exploration of the Sea C.M.* 1967/E:1–7.

Elston, R.A. 1988. *Bonamia ostreae* disease of European flat oyster (*Ostrea edulis*) in North America: Occurrence, environmental effects and host range (abstract). *Journal of Shellfish Research* 7(1):116–117.

FAO (Food and Agriculture Organization of the United Nations). 2004. Surveillance and zoning for aquatic animal diseases. *In* R.P. Subasinghe, S.E. McGladdery, and B.J. Hill, editors. FAO Fisheries Technical Paper No. 451. Fisheries and Agriculture Organization, Rome, Italy. 73 pp.

FAO/NACA (Food and Agriculture Organization of the United Nations/Network of Aquaculture Centres in Asia–Pacific). 2000. *Asia Regional Technical Guidelines on Health Management for the Responsible Movement of Live Aquatic Animals and the Beijing Consensus and Implementation Strategy*. FAO Fisheries Technical Paper No. 402. Fisheries and Agriculture Organization, Rome, Italy. On-line version, www.enaca.org/NACA-Publications/AsiaRegionalTechnicalGuidelines.pdf.

FAO/NACA (Food and Agriculture Organization of the United Nations/Network of Aquaculture Centres in Asia–Pacific). 2001. *Manual of Procedures for the Implementation of the Asia Regional Technical Guidelines on Health Management for the Responsible Movement of Live Aquatic Animals*. FAO Fisheries Technical Paper No. 402/1. Fisheries and Agriculture Organization, Rome, Italy. On-line version, www.enaca.org/NACA-Publications/Manual-of-Procedures.pdf.

Found, H.R. and R.R. Logie. 1957. *Rehabilitation of Disease-Depleted Oyster Fisheries*. Fisheries Research Board of Canada, General Series Circular No. 29, Biological Station of St. Andrews, New Brunswick, April 1959. 2 pp.

Garrett, L. 1995. *The Coming Plague: Newly Emerging Diseases in a World Out of Balance*. Penguin Books, London, UK. 768 pp.

Hervio, D., S.M. Bower, and G.R. Meyer. 1996. Detection, isolation and experimental transmission of *Mikrocytos mackini*, a microcell parasite of Pacific oysters *Crassostrea gigas*. *Journal of Invertebrate Pathology* 67:72–79.

Hine, P.M., S.M. Bower, G.R. Meyer, N. Cochennec-Laureau, and F.C.J. Berthe. 2001. Ultrastructure of *Mikrocytos mackini*, the cause of Denman Island Disease in oysters *Crassostrea* spp. and *Ostrea* spp. in British Columbia, Canada. *Diseases of Aquatic Organisms* 45:215–227.

ICES (International Council for the Exploration of the Seas). 1984. *Guidelines for Implementing the ICES Code of Practice Concerning Introductions and Transfers of Marine and Freshwater Organisms*. Cooperative Research Report No. 130. ICES, Copenhagen, Denmark. 12 pp.

ICES (International Council for the Exploration of the Seas). 1988. *Codes of Practice and Manual of Procedures for Consideration of the Introductions and Transfers of Marine and Freshwater Organisms*. *In* G.E. Turner, editor. Cooperative Research Report No. 159 (prepared jointly with

the European Inland Fisheries Advisory Council [EIFAC] and published as EIFAC Occasional Paper No. 23, 44 pp., 1988).

ICES (International Council for the Exploration of the Seas). 1995. *ICES Code of Practice on the Introductions and Transfers of Marine Organisms—1994*. Annex III to ICES Co-operative Research Report No. 204. ICES, Copenhagen, Denmark. 17 pp.

ICES (International Council for the Exploration of the Seas). 2003. *Code of Practice on the Introductions and Transfers of Marine Organisms*. ICES, Copenhagen, Denmark. On-line version, http://www.ices.dk/pubs/itmo.pdf.

Joly, J.-P., S.M. Bower, and G.R. Meyer. 2001. A simple technique to concentrate the protozoan *Mikrocytos mackini*, causative agent of Denman Island disease in oysters. *The Journal of Parasitology* 87:432–434.

Karlsson, J.D. 1991. Parasites of the bay scallop, *Argopecten irradians* (Lamarck, 1819). Pages 180–190 *in* S.E. Shumway and P.A. Sandifer, editors. *International Compendium of Scallop Biology and Culture*. World Aquaculture Society and National Shellfisheries Association, Baton Rouge, LA.

Lee, C.-S. and P.J. O'Bryen, editors. 2003. *Biosecurity in Aquaculture Production Systems: Exclusion of Pathogens and Other Undesirables*. The World Aquaculture Society, Baton Rouge, LA. 293 pp.

Li, M.F., G.S. Traxler, S. Clyburne, and J.E. Stewart. 1980. Malpeque disease, isolation and morphology of a *Labyrinthomyxa*-like organism from diseased oysters. *International Council for the Exploration of the Sea C.M.* 1980/F(15):1–9.

Litvak, M.K. 1999. The development of winter flounder (*Pleuronectes americanus*) for aquaculture in Atlantic Canada: Current status and future prospects. *Aquaculture* 176:55–64.

Martin-Robichaud, D.J. 2003. Haddock broodstock management. Pages 17–22 *in* D.E. Aiken, editor. *Early Rearing of Haddock: State of the Art*. Proceedings of the Workshop: 16–17 October 2002, St. Andrews, New Brunswick Canada. Aquaculture Association of Canada Special Publication No. 7. pp. 17–22.

McGladdery, S.E. and S.M. Bower. 1999. *Synopsis of Infectious Diseases and Parasites of Commercially Exploited Shellfish: Malpeque Disease of Oysters*. Fisheries and Oceans Canada-Pacific Region. On-line version, http://www-sci.pac.dfo-mpo.gc.ca/shelldis/pages/maldisoy_e.htm.

McGladdery, S.E., B.C. Bradford, and D.J. Scarratt. 1993. Investigations into transmission of parasites of bay scallop, *Argopecten irradians* (Lamarck, 1819) during quarantine introduction into Canadian waters. *Journal of Shellfish Research* 12:49–58.

McGladdery, S.E. and M.F. Stephenson. 1999. Malpeque disease of American oysters (*Crassostrea virginica*)—Transmission experiment results (abstract). Page 8 *in Proceedings of the 9th International Conference of the European Association of Fish Pathologists*. 19–14 September 1999, Rhodes, Greece.

Needler, A.W.H. and R.R. Logie. 1947. Serious mortalities in Prince Edward Island oysters caused by a contagious disease. *Transactions of the Royal Society of Canada XLI(III)*Section V: 73–89.

Nielsen, O., A. Clavijo and J.A. Boughen. 2001b. Serologic evidence of influenza A infection in marine mammals of Arctic Canada. *Journal of Wildlife Diseases* 37(4):820–825.

Nielsen, O., R.E.A. Stewart, K. Nielsen, L. Measures, and P. Duignan. 2001a. Serologic survey of *Brucella* spp. antibodies in some marine mammals of North America. *Journal of Wildlife Diseases* 37,(1):89–100.

OIE (World Organisation for Animal Health). 2003. *Manual of Diagnostic Tests for Aquatic Animals*, 4th edition. Office International des Epizooties, Paris, France. 358 pp. On-line version, www.oie.int.

OIE (World Organisation for Animal Health). 2004. *Aquatic Animal Health Code*, 7th edition. Office International des Epizooties, Paris, France. 167 pp. On-line version, www.oie.int.

Quayle, D.B. 1961. *Denman Island disease and mortality, 1960*. Fisheries Research Board of Canada Manuscript Report No. 713. Fisheries and Oceans Canada, Ottawa, Ontario, Canada.

Ragone-Calvo, L.M., G.W. Calvo, and E.M. Burreson. 2003. Dual disease resistance in selectively bred eastern oyster, *Crassostrea virginica*, strain tested in Chesapeake Bay. *Aquaculture* 220(1–4):69–82.

Sindermann, C.J. 1956. Diseases of fishes in the western Atlantic. IV. Fungus disease and resultant mortalities of herring in the Gulf of St. Lawrence in 1955. Maine Department of Sea and Shore Fisheries, *Research Bulletin* 25:1–23.

Stephenson, M.F. and S.E. McGladdery. 2002. Detection of a previously undescribed Haplosporidian-like infection of a blue mussel (*Mytilus edulis*) in Atlantic Canada (abstract). *Journal of Shellfish Research* 21(1):389.

Stephenson, M.F., S.E. McGladdery, M. Maillet, A. Veniot, and G. Meyer. 2003. First reported occurrence of MSX in Canada (abstract). *Journal of Shellfish Research* 22(1):355.

Walker, P. and R.P. Subasinghe, editors. 2000. *DNA-Based Molecular Diagnostic Techniques: Research Needs for Standardization and Validation of the Detection of Aquatic Animal Pathogens and Diseases*. FAO (Food and Agriculture Organization of the United Nations) Fisheries Technical Paper No. 395. FAO, Rome, Italy. 93 pp.

Whyte, S.K., R.J. Cawthorn, S.E. McGladdery, and R.J. MacMillan. 1993. Cross-transmission studies of *Perkinsus karlssoni* (Apicomplexa) from bay scallops *Argopecten irradians* to native Atlantic Canadian shellfish species. *Diseases of Aquatic Organisms* 17(1):33–39.

Whyte, S.K., R.J. Cawthorn, and S.E. McGladdery. 1994. Co-infection of bay scallops, *Argopecten irradians*, with *Perkinsus karlssoni* (Apicomplexa, Perkinsea) and an unidentified coccidian parasite (Apicomplexa) in the bay scallop *Argopecten irradians*. *Diseases of Aquatic Organisms* 18:53–62.

Wosniok, W., T. Lang, V. Dethlefsen, S.W. Fiest, A.H. McVicar, S. Mellergaard, and A.D. Vethaak, editors. 2000. Analysis of ICES long-term data on disease of North Sea dab (*Limanda limanda*) in relation to contaminants and other environmental factors. *International Council for the Exploration of the Sea C.M.* 2000/S:12, 15.

WTO (World Trade Organization). 2004. *The WTO Agreement on the Application of Sanitary and Phytosanitary Measures (SPS Agreement)*. World Trade Organization, Geneva, Switzerland. Online version, www.wto.org/english/tratop_e/sps_e/spsagr_e.htm.

Chapter 5

The U.S. Fish & Wildlife Service's "Aquatic Animal Health Policy": Innovative Approaches to Managing Diseases in Traditional and Special-Case Aquatic Animals

Thomas A. Bell, J. Scott Foott, Kathy Clemens, Susan Gutenberger, Ray Brunson, John Thoesen, Rick Nelson, Norm Heil, John Coll, and Crystal Hudson

Abstract

The U.S. Fish & Wildlife Service recently revised its internal "Fish Health Policy" chapters in the Service's *Manual*. The chapters are now referred to as the "Aquatic Animal Health Policy" (AAHP), as the Service now holds and rears a greater number of species within the National Fish Hatchery System, including non-finfish. Potentially accompanying this increased diversity of species may be new aquatic animal pathogens of which little are known. Additionally, many of these new pathogens have yet to be discovered.

The new AAHP has been extensively reviewed within the Service, and by agencies and organizations outside of the Service. The AAHP was developed to (a) be more readily adaptable to current needs and (b) address animal health risk-assessment needs relative to "new" and little-understood species under care of the Service.

In addition, the AAHP contains a new chapter dedicated to newly developed animal health risk-assessment tools designed specifically to assist resource managers in minimizing the health risks associated with the movement of special-case aquatic species (e.g., threatened and endangered species) onto and off of the U.S. Fish and Wildlife Service facilities. To make the best decisions possible relative to the U.S. aquatic resources, resource managers must first be equipped with information soundly based on facts and high-confidence-level scientific opinions. These new tools allow aquatic animal health professionals to (a) proactively inform resource managers of the level of risk

Thomas A. Bell, corresponding author. E-mail: thomas_a_bell@fws.gov

associated with imminent aquatic animal movements, especially those of special-case animals and (b) recommend means to mitigate or remove risks associated with such animal movements.

Introduction

The U.S. Fish & Wildlife Service's (Service) Division of the National Fish Hatchery System (NFHS) maintains 86 facilities, including 69 national fish hatcheries (NFHs), one historic hatchery, nine fish health centers (FHCs), six fish technology centers (FTCs), and the office of the Aquatic Animal Drug Approval Partnership Program. The facilities are scattered throughout the contiguous 48 states. The NFHS serves the American public by providing fish and other aquatic species for several purposes. The NFHS is part of the Service's Fisheries program, whose objectives are to recover listed (i.e., threatened or endangered) and candidate aquatic species, restore depleted aquatic populations to preclude their being listed as threatened or endangered, manage fisheries that fall under the purview of more than one jurisdiction (i.e., interjurisdictional), restore interjurisdictional fisheries and aquatic ecosystems, mitigate impacts from Federal water projects, and provide fish and wildlife management assistance to tribes and on Service lands.

The health of the aquatic animals being reared and held at NFHS facilities is vital to the success of its programs. The Service's FHCs and FTCs are essential elements in meeting that need. Key to maintaining a high level of fitness within the animal populations on Service facilities is a robust system of health monitoring and disease prevention. The Service has a history, since the 1970s, of operating under a predefined set of "standard operating procedures," which have been referred to as the "Fish Health Policy," and comprise several chapters within the *U.S. Fish & Wildlife Service Manual.*

The Fish Health Policy (Policy), by definition, serves as the basis for efforts to contain, control, and minimize the impacts of aquatic animal pathogens and diseases on Service-managed and Service-contracted properties, and the U.S. natural resources. In response to requirements to hold and rear an increasingly diverse variety of aquatic species (including species other than finfish), the Service has revised the Policy. To reflect that diversity, the Policy has been renamed the Aquatic Animal Health Policy (AAHP). The Policy is publicly accessible online at http://policy.fws.gov/ser700.html.

The Policy was also modified to make it more flexible to allow for future revisions. This was achieved by moving all of the technical/scientific methods and procedures from the Policy to the newly created *U.S. Fish & Wildlife Service Handbook of Aquatic Animal Health Procedures and Protocols* (parts of which were jointly developed and published with the American Fisheries Society's Fish Health Section). Administratively, the *Handbook* does not require the same level of review, and can thus be readily changed as protocols for disease detection improve. The *Handbook* is the all-inclusive documentation of standard procedures/techniques by the Service and is available online at http://policy.fws.gov/713hb.html.

Biosecurity and the Service's Aquatic Animal Health Policy

Biosecurity is extremely germane to the current programmatic needs of the Service. A high level of concern about the unintentional movement of pathogens on to and/or off of a

Service facilities resulted in the addition of a completely new chapter to the AAHP. The new chapter, "Special Case Aquatic Animal Movements and Controlled Propagation Programs," is focused on newly developed animal-health risk-assessment tools. The explicit purpose of the chapter is to provide guidelines for the generation of fish health recommendations to Service facilities and personnel involved in the movement and rearing of special-case aquatic animals.

To make the best decisions possible relative to the U.S. aquatic resources, resource managers must first be equipped with information soundly based on facts and high-confidence-level scientific opinions. These new tools allow aquatic animal health professionals to (a) proactively inform resource managers of the risk associated with imminent aquatic animal movements (especially those of special-case animals) via a consistent, thorough, and nationally uniform document and (b) recommend means to mitigate or remove fish health risks associated with such animal movements.

As noted earlier, the Service is being increasingly asked to hold and/or rear aquatic animals for which there is little, if any, knowledge on the animal's life cycle, rearing techniques, normally occurring pathogens, or other information needed to rear the animals in captivity. In spite of the paucity of information about these new species, a decision must be made relative to moving them on to and/or off of a Service facility, and the decision must often be made very quickly (e.g., the watershed for a listed species is drying up due to a severe drought). Even if a manager has never seen this species before, he or she must decide if (a) these animals pose a health risk to existing stocks on the facility, (b) existing stocks pose a health risk to the new species, (c) returning them to a watershed will jeopardize their health status, or (d) returning them to a watershed will be futile, because of an endemic pathogen that could seriously harm or eliminate the "new" species.

The new AAHP chapter, "Special Case Aquatic Animal Movements and Controlled Propagation Programs," contains two worksheets. These worksheets, to be completed prior to any movement of special-case species, compel the Service fish health professional (in consultation with appropriate resource managers, partners, and facilities, i.e., the review team) to systematically examine potential risk components that should be factored into a recommendation regarding the relative health risk of the planned movement. In addition to allowing the fish health professional to assign a risk factor to such a movement, the new chapter also provides guidance on recommended measures to mitigate or eliminate the estimated risk.

Risk-assessment worksheets

Worksheet for animal movements into a Service facility

All special-case aquatic animal movements into a Service facility must be preceded by a Service fish health professional (and review team) providing recommendations to the facility manager relative to the health risks and means to mitigate or eliminate these risks. To aid in making these recommendations, the fish health professional (and review team) will complete FWS Form 3-2261, "Considerations or Factors Relative to Movements into a Facility" (Table 5.1).

The form leads the Service fish health professional (and review team) through a series of questions and associated responses addressing the following factors: type of animal,

Table 5.1 Considerations or factors relative to movements into a facility, modified from USFWS Form 3-2261, 11/03 (USFWS 2003c)

Consideration or factor (factor weight)	Response value	Factor score
Animal (5)		
Traditional aquaculture species (1)	–	–
Non-traditional species (5)	–	
Lifestage (10)		
Gametes/fertilized eggs with parental history of no significant pathogens (1)	–	–
Gametes/fertilized eggs with parental history of significant pathogens (5)	–	
Gametes/fertilized eggs with no parental history (5)	–	
Animal (5)	–	
Receiving facility location (5)		
Within propagated population's watershed (2)	–	–
Outside of propagated population's watershed (5)	–	
Pathogen surveillance of proposed propagated feral population or related populations in same watershed (10)		
High level of population pathogen history (multiple, statistically valid, and lethal samples)		
Significant pathogen(s) of concern detected (5)	–	–
No significant pathogens detected (1)	–	
Low level of population pathogen history (single and/or non-standard samples)		
Significant pathogen(s) of concern detected (5)	–	–
No significant pathogens detected (3)	–	
No population pathogen history (5)	–	
Facility disease history (10)		
High level of facility pathogen history (multiple, statistically valid, and lethal samples)		
Significant pathogen(s) of concern detected (5)	–	–
No significant pathogens detected (1)	–	
Low level of facility pathogen history (single and/or non-standard samples)		
Significant pathogen(s) of concern detected (5)	–	–
No significant pathogens detected (3)	–	
No facility pathogen history (5)	–	
Facility health capabilities (diagnostics and sampling) (1)		
High (diagnostic and sampling capabilities) (1)	–	–
Medium (sampling capabilities) (3)	–	
Low (require on-site FHC assistance) (5)	–	
Facility type (10)		
Isolation A/quarantine (as defined in 713 FW 1 and 5) (1)	–	–
Isolation B (as defined in 713 FW 1 and 5) (2)	–	
Isolation C (as defined in 713 FW 1 and 5) (3)	–	
Intensive (high environmental control) (5)	–	
Extensive (low environmental control) (7)	–	
Water source (5)		
Closed (protected or enclosed well or spring) (1)	–	–
Open, animal free or treated/disinfected (2)	–	
Open, with any animals (non-treated or non-disinfected) (5)	–	

Table 5.1 (*Continued*)

Consideration or factor (factor weight)	Response value	Factor score
Cultural impacts on animal health (knowledge of requirements for species) (5)		
Optimal (understand cultural requirements) (1)	_	_
Adequate (incomplete cultural requirements understood) (3)	_	
Unknown (automatically pick "unknown" under facilities) (5)	_	
Cultural impacts on animal health (facilities) (10)		
Optimal (minimal stress for growth, reproduction, or etc.) (1)	_	_
Adequate (for maintenance, potential health problems) (3)	_	
Inadequate (high probability of significant mortalities) (5)	_	
Unknown (due to "unknown" cultural requirements) (5)	_	
Total risk score		_

Note: The form is completed by a fish health professional and provided as part of an animal health risk-assessment for movement of aquatic species onto a facility. The factor score for each major factor is obtained by multiplying the factor weight (number in parentheses after the factor, e.g., "Animal" has a factor weight of 5) by the response value (number in parentheses after the chosen response, e.g., "traditional aquaculture species" has a value of 1). The total risk score is the sum of all factor scores.

Table 5.2 Risk classification and isolation recommendations for aquatic animals moving onto facilities based on health risk scores. Excerpted from USFWS (2003a)

Health risk score	Risk classification	Recommended isolation level
250–376	High	Level A—quarantine for entire rearing cycle
150–249	Moderate	Level B—restricted rearing conditions for a defined period to allow for testing
<150	Low	Level C—standard intensive, extensive

Note: Health risk scores generated using the form shown in Table 5.1 can be converted to a "risk classification," with associated recommendations relative to isolation needed to mitigate the calculated risk.

life-stage being moved, location of receiving facility, history of pathogen surveillance within the population being moved, disease history of the receiving facility, animal health expertise at the receiving facility, type of receiving facility, water source for the facility, rearing practices knowledge-base, and impact of that knowledge-base.

Each of the above factors has been assigned a weighted value based on its relative importance when compared with the other factors. Under each factor, there are at least two answers/responses from which to choose. Each answer in turn has been assigned a numeric value. A "factor score" is obtained by multiplying the topic-weighted value by the answer value. The sum total of all ten factor scores is referred to as the "total risk score."

The total risk score is then compared to values on an associated table (Table 5.2), "Risk Classification and Isolation Recommendations for Aquatic Animals Moving onto Facilities, Based on Health Risk Scores."

The total risk score can be converted into a "Risk Classification" (i.e., high, moderate, or low risk) from which the fish health professional (and review team) can recommend the level of isolation required to minimize (or eliminate) the estimated risk.

Worksheet for animal movements from a Service facility

The process for assessing the health risk relative to animal movements from a Service facility is nearly identical to that for animals moving onto a Service facility. As in the "onto a Service facility" situation, a Service fish health professional (and review team) will complete a similar form, FWS Form 3-2262, "Considerations or Factors Relative to Movements from a Facility" (Table 5.3).

This form comprises only five factors for consideration. These include: confidence level of the surveillance methods used to assess pathogen status in the receiving watershed, confidence level of the degree of surveillance and the number of animals examined in the receiving watershed, life-stage and parental history of animals to be released, level of pathogen surveillance within the population being released, and relationship of the receiving watershed to that of the Service facility and the original watershed of the population.

In exactly the same fashion as that for animals moving onto a facility, a "factor score" is derived by multiplying the factor's weighted value by the value assigned to the answer chosen. The composite value of all factor scores is equal to the total risk score. The total risk score is then compared to values on an associated table (Table 5.4), "Risk Classification and Isolation Recommendations for Aquatic Animals Moving Off of Facilities Based on Health Risk Scores." The Total Risk Score can be converted into a "Risk Classification" (i.e., high, moderate, or low risk), from which the fish health professional (and review team) can make recommendations for movement of animals based on inherent animal health risks.

Worksheet examples

Several hypothetical examples for the use of the risk-assessment worksheets are offered.

Movement of animals into a Service facility

Wild rainbow trout (*Oncorhynchus mykiss*) adults are captured and spawned in the resident stream. Iodophor-treated eggs are sent to the isolation building at the Service's "Timbuktu" National Fish Hatchery (Level B, well water, no effluent disinfection; see Table 5.5). The hatchery is not in the same watershed as the resident stream. There is no disease history for the trout population. The "Timbuktu" NFH, however, has had an *Aeromonas salmonicida* problem for the past 3 years.

The resulting health risk score for this situation is 221 (Table 5.6). The health risk score equates to a moderate risk classification (Table 5.2). The hatchery manager and others involved in the planned move would be informed of the inherent risk of the movement. The current hatchery has a Level B isolation status, and is therefore adequate to rear the trout. To decrease the risk, however, to the subject trout population and the resident populations already on the facility, the hatchery could add a disinfection system to their isolation unit effluent. This would increase their isolation unit status to Level A, and would further reduce the associated health risk.

Table 5.3 Considerations or factors relative to movements from a facility, modified from USFWS Form 3-2262, 11/03 (USFWS 2003d)

Consideration or factor (factor weight)	Response value	Factor score
Confidence of pathogen surveillance—Methods (5)		
Standard methods (includes lethal) as per Section A of the *Handbook* (1)	–	–
Non-traditional methods (e.g., NWFHS Section C from the *Handbook*) (3)	–	
No surveillance conducted (7)	–	
Confidence of pathogen surveillance—Efforts (5)		
No surveillance conducted (0)	–	–
Standard inspection (includes lethal) to include examination of representative sample of moribund animals (1)	–	
Examination of non-representative sample of animals (4)	–	
Lifestage released (5)		
Gametes/fertilized eggs with parental history of no significant pathogens (1)	–	–
Gametes/fertilized eggs with parental history of significant pathogens (5)	–	
Gametes/fertilized eggs with no parental history (5)	–	
Animal (5)	–	
Pathogen surveillance of proposed propagated population (10)		
High level of population pathogen history (multiple, statistically valid, and lethal samples)		
Significant pathogen(s) detected in population and not known in receiving watershed (5)	–	–
Significant pathogen(s) detected in population and present in receiving watershed (3)	–	
No significant pathogens detected (1)	–	
Low level of population pathogen history (single and/or non-standard samples)	–	–
Significant pathogen(s) detected in population and not known in receiving watershed (5)		
Significant pathogen(s) detected in population and present in receiving watershed (3)	–	
No significant pathogens detected (3)	–	
No population pathogen history (5)	–	
Receiving watershed (20)		
Same as propagated population's original watershed and facility's watershed (1)	–	–
Same as population's original watershed, not facility's watershed, and closed water supply (1)	–	
Same as population's original watershed, not facility's watershed, and open water supply (3)	–	
Different from population's original watershed and same as facility's (3)	–	
Different from propagated population's original watershed and different from facility's watershed (5)	–	
Total risk score		

Note: Each factor score is obtained by multiplying the factor weight (number in parentheses after the major factor, e.g., "lifestage released" has a factor weight of 5) by the response value (number in parentheses after the chosen response, e.g., "Animal" has a response value of 5). The total risk score is the sum of all the factor scores, and can be converted to a "risk classification" and associated recommendations by using the values shown in Table 5.4.

Table 5.4 Risk classification and isolation recommendations for aquatic animals moving off of facilities based on health risk scores. Excerpted from USFWS (2003b)

Health risk score	Risk classification	Recommended movement
125–175	High	None. Movement to another isolation facility or to waters of origin
81–124	Moderate	Only that restricted to facilities or waters that have written approval of attending FHCD
<80	Low	Unrestricted movement out of isolation

Note: Health risk scores generated using the form shown in Table 5.3 can be converted to a "risk classification," with associated recommendations relative to type of movement consistent with mitigation of the calculated risk.

Table 5.5 Description of isolation level classifications and definition of associated terms. Excerpted from USFWS (2004)

Isolation level or term	Isolation conditions or definition of term
Isolation level "A"	*A quarantine facility with the following characteristics*: • Completely enclosed, locked structure with a given room or space allotted to only one Captive Propagation Program (CPP) population. Water is supplied by either a well or is disinfected (ozone/ultraviolet light). • Operated, by a written standard operating plan, with the highest level of sanitation, including, but not limited to, restricted personnel access; dedicated equipment, such as brooms, nets, etc.; dedicated external garments, such as boots and rain gear; disinfection foot baths; and landfill disposal of carcasses. • Effluent is disinfected by ultraviolet light sterilization or strong oxidation (i.e., chlorination system recommended, see *Handbook*), or is sent into a documented "dead-end" location that cannot enter facility water supplies or receiving waters (e.g., leach field distant from facility).
Isolation level "B"	Same as Level A, except effluent is not disinfected prior to contact with a receiving watershed. Effluent from this facility should not contact any water supplies at the facility.
Isolation level "C"	Same as Level B, except multiple populations or groups may be housed in the same containment building, and there is no restriction on the facility water supply. It is recommended that some form of airborne pathogen separation between populations (such as curtains), as well as unit-specific equipment, be used in this type facility.
Intensive-culture facility	Open facility with adjacent rearing units that allow for direct observation and husbandry of CPP species (e.g., standard hatchery with raceways and tanks). Typically, animal densities are high, and rearing units are in proximity to each other.
Extensive-culture facility	Open facility with limited ability for observation and husbandry of CPP species (e.g., earthen pond systems). Typically, animal densities are low to moderate, and rearing units are not in close proximity to each other.

Table 5.6 Example completed risk-assessment worksheet for the hypothetical movement of rainbow trout onto a hypothetical facility

Consideration or factor (factor weight)	Response value	Factor score
Animal (5)		
Traditional aquaculture species (1)	1	5
Non-traditional species (5)	–	
Lifestage (10)		
Gametes/fertilized eggs with parental history of no significant pathogens (1)	–	50
Gametes/fertilized eggs with parental history of significant pathogens (5)	–	
Gametes/fertilized eggs with no parental history (5)	5	
Animal (5)	–	
Receiving facility location (5)		
Within propagated population's watershed (2)	–	25
Outside of propagated population's watershed (5)	5	
Pathogen surveillance of proposed propagated feral population or related populations in same watershed (10)		
High level of population pathogen history (multiple, statistically valid, and lethal samples)		
Significant pathogen(s) of concern detected (5)	–	na
No significant pathogens detected (1)	–	
Low level of population pathogen history (single and/or non-standard samples)		
Significant pathogen(s) of concern detected (5)	–	50
No significant pathogens detected (3)	–	
No population pathogen history (5)	5	
Facility disease history (10)		
High level of facility pathogen history (multiple, statistically valid, and lethal samples)		
Significant pathogen(s) of concern detected (5)	5	50
No significant pathogens detected (1)	–	
Low level of facility pathogen history (single and/or non-standard samples)		
Significant pathogen(s) of concern detected (5)	–	na
No significant pathogens detected (3)	–	
No facility pathogen history (5)	–	
Facility health capabilities (diagnostics and sampling) (1)		
High (diagnostic and sampling capabilities) (1)	1	1
Medium (sampling capabilities) (3)	–	
Low (require on-site FHC assistance) (5)	–	
Facility type (10)		
Isolation A/quarantine (as defined in 713 FW 1 and 5) (1)	–	20
Isolation B (as defined in 713 FW 1 and 5) (2)	2	
Isolation C (as defined in 713 FW 1 and 5) (3)	–	
Intensive (high environmental control) (5)	–	
Extensive (low environmental control) (7)	–	
Water source (5)		
Closed (protected or enclosed well or spring) (1)	1	5
Open, animal free or treated/disinfected (2)	–	
Open, with any animals (non-treated or non-disinfected) (5)	–	
Cultural impacts on animal health (knowledge of requirements for species) (5)		
Optimal (understand cultural requirements) (1)	1	5
Adequate (incomplete cultural requirements understood) (3)	–	
Unknown (automatically pick "unknown" under facilities) (5)	–	

(Continues)

Table 5.6 (*Continued*)

Consideration or factor (factor weight)	Response value	Factor score
Cultural impacts on animal health (facilities) (10)		
Optimal (minimal stress for growth, reproduction, or etc.) (1)	1	10
Adequate (for maintenance, potential health problems) (3)	–	
Inadequate (high probability of significant mortalities) (5)	–	
Unknown (due to "unknown" cultural requirements) (5)	–	
Total risk score		221

Note: The total risk score can be converted to a "risk classification" and associated recommendations by using the values shown in Table 5.2. This example represents a moderate risk classification.

Movement of animals into a Service facility

A non-Service cooperator has been contracted by the Service (i.e., facilities contracted by the Service are considered, in the context of the AAHP, to be Service facilities) to capture larval big-lipped crayfish (imaginary species) and rear them in a pond adjacent to their natal stream. This Service cooperator also maintains other finfish and crustaceans within different ponds on the same facility. The source water for the pond is the natal stream of the crayfish and has a 6.35 mm (0.25 in) screen, as does the effluent, which is returned directly to the same stream. No one has ever attempted to culture this endangered species before, and very little is known of its life cycle. Additionally, no studies have been conducted to assess its typical pathogen load. The big-lipped crayfish is not only endangered, but its watershed (the only one it occupies, due to unique water characteristics) is scheduled to be reduced to approximately 10% of normal flow due to hydroelectric-related changes upstream.

The resulting health risk score for this situation is 360 (Table 5.7). The health risk score equates to a high-risk classification (Table 5.2). The hatchery manager and others involved in the planned move would be informed of the inherent high risk of the movement. In this case, the isolation capabilities of the hatchery are non-existent, and are thus equivalent to or less than Level C status (see Table 5.5). Because the animals are on the Federal Endangered Species list, their health, once on site, is paramount. To reduce the threats to the safety of these aquatic animals, the fish health professional (and review team) would recommend that significant modifications be made to minimize the risk to the subject crayfish population and the other aquatic animal population(s) already on the facility. The hatchery manager, as well as other Service professionals, would have to weigh these "costs of safety" against the importance of an endangered species being saved from possible extinction.

Movement of animals from a Service facility

The "Transylvania" Fish Technology Center (TFTC) has successfully reared purple sturgeon (imaginary species) in tanks for 5 years in a well-water facility. The TFTC is located outside of the natural range of the sturgeon. Effluent from the facility is discharged into a city sewer system, and any mortalities that might occur will go to the local landfill. During the 5-year rearing period, no significant pathogens have been detected in the captive population, based on three inspections performed as outlined in the Service's *Handbook*. It is proposed that

Table 5.6 Example completed risk-assessment worksheet for the hypothetical movement of rainbow trout onto a hypothetical facility

Consideration or factor (factor weight)	Response value	Factor score
Animal (5)		
Traditional aquaculture species (1)	1	5
Non-traditional species (5)	–	
Lifestage (10)		
Gametes/fertilized eggs with parental history of no significant pathogens (1)	–	50
Gametes/fertilized eggs with parental history of significant pathogens (5)	–	
Gametes/fertilized eggs with no parental history (5)	5	
Animal (5)	–	
Receiving facility location (5)		
Within propagated population's watershed (2)	–	25
Outside of propagated population's watershed (5)	5	
Pathogen surveillance of proposed propagated feral population or related populations in same watershed (10)		
High level of population pathogen history (multiple, statistically valid, and lethal samples)		
Significant pathogen(s) of concern detected (5)	–	na
No significant pathogens detected (1)	–	
Low level of population pathogen history (single and/or non-standard samples)		
Significant pathogen(s) of concern detected (5)	–	50
No significant pathogens detected (3)	–	
No population pathogen history (5)	5	
Facility disease history (10)		
High level of facility pathogen history (multiple, statistically valid, and lethal samples)		
Significant pathogen(s) of concern detected (5)	5	50
No significant pathogens detected (1)	–	
Low level of facility pathogen history (single and/or non-standard samples)		
Significant pathogen(s) of concern detected (5)	–	na
No significant pathogens detected (3)	–	
No facility pathogen history (5)	–	
Facility health capabilities (diagnostics and sampling) (1)		
High (diagnostic and sampling capabilities) (1)	1	1
Medium (sampling capabilities) (3)	–	
Low (require on-site FHC assistance) (5)	–	
Facility type (10)		
Isolation A/quarantine (as defined in 713 FW 1 and 5) (1)	–	20
Isolation B (as defined in 713 FW 1 and 5) (2)	2	
Isolation C (as defined in 713 FW 1 and 5) (3)	–	
Intensive (high environmental control) (5)	–	
Extensive (low environmental control) (7)	–	
Water source (5)		
Closed (protected or enclosed well or spring) (1)	1	5
Open, animal free or treated/disinfected (2)	–	
Open, with any animals (non-treated or non-disinfected) (5)	–	
Cultural impacts on animal health (knowledge of requirements for species) (5)		
Optimal (understand cultural requirements) (1)	1	5
Adequate (incomplete cultural requirements understood) (3)	–	
Unknown (automatically pick "unknown" under facilities) (5)	–	

(*Continues*)

Table 5.6 (*Continued*)

Consideration or factor (factor weight)	Response value	Factor score
Cultural impacts on animal health (facilities) (10)		
Optimal (minimal stress for growth, reproduction, or etc.) (1)	1	10
Adequate (for maintenance, potential health problems) (3)	–	
Inadequate (high probability of significant mortalities) (5)	–	
Unknown (due to "unknown" cultural requirements) (5)	–	
Total risk score		221

Note: The total risk score can be converted to a "risk classification" and associated recommendations by using the values shown in Table 5.2. This example represents a moderate risk classification.

Movement of animals into a Service facility

A non-Service cooperator has been contracted by the Service (i.e., facilities contracted by the Service are considered, in the context of the AAHP, to be Service facilities) to capture larval big-lipped crayfish (imaginary species) and rear them in a pond adjacent to their natal stream. This Service cooperator also maintains other finfish and crustaceans within different ponds on the same facility. The source water for the pond is the natal stream of the crayfish and has a 6.35 mm (0.25 in) screen, as does the effluent, which is returned directly to the same stream. No one has ever attempted to culture this endangered species before, and very little is known of its life cycle. Additionally, no studies have been conducted to assess its typical pathogen load. The big-lipped crayfish is not only endangered, but its watershed (the only one it occupies, due to unique water characteristics) is scheduled to be reduced to approximately 10% of normal flow due to hydroelectric-related changes upstream.

The resulting health risk score for this situation is 360 (Table 5.7). The health risk score equates to a high-risk classification (Table 5.2). The hatchery manager and others involved in the planned move would be informed of the inherent high risk of the movement. In this case, the isolation capabilities of the hatchery are non-existent, and are thus equivalent to or less than Level C status (see Table 5.5). Because the animals are on the Federal Endangered Species list, their health, once on site, is paramount. To reduce the threats to the safety of these aquatic animals, the fish health professional (and review team) would recommend that significant modifications be made to minimize the risk to the subject crayfish population and the other aquatic animal population(s) already on the facility. The hatchery manager, as well as other Service professionals, would have to weigh these "costs of safety" against the importance of an endangered species being saved from possible extinction.

Movement of animals from a Service facility

The "Transylvania" Fish Technology Center (TFTC) has successfully reared purple sturgeon (imaginary species) in tanks for 5 years in a well-water facility. The TFTC is located outside of the natural range of the sturgeon. Effluent from the facility is discharged into a city sewer system, and any mortalities that might occur will go to the local landfill. During the 5-year rearing period, no significant pathogens have been detected in the captive population, based on three inspections performed as outlined in the Service's *Handbook*. It is proposed that

Table 5.7 Example completed risk-assessment worksheet for the movement of a hypothetical species, the big-lipped crayfish, onto a facility. This example represents a high-risk classification

Factor	Response value	Factor score
Animal (5)		
Traditional aquaculture species (1)	–	25
Non-traditional species (5)	5	
Lifestage (10)		
Gametes/fertilized eggs with parental history of no significant pathogens (1)	–	50
Gametes/fertilized eggs with parental history of significant pathogens (5)	–	
Gametes/fertilized eggs with no parental history (5)	–	
Animal (5)	5	
Receiving facility location (5)		
Within propagated population's watershed (2)	2	10
Outside of propagated population's watershed (5)	–	
Pathogen surveillance of proposed propagated feral population or related populations in same watershed (10)		
High level of population pathogen history (multiple, statistically valid, and lethal samples)		
Significant pathogen(s) of concern detected (5)	–	Na
No significant pathogens detected (1)	–	
Low level of population pathogen history (single and/or non-standard samples)		
Significant pathogen(s) of concern detected (5)	–	50
No significant pathogens detected (3)	–	
No population pathogen history (5)	5	
Facility disease history (10)		
High level of facility pathogen history (multiple, statistically valid, and lethal samples)		
Significant pathogen(s) of concern detected (5)	–	Na
No significant pathogens detected (1)	–	
Low level of facility pathogen history (single and/or non-standard samples)		
Significant pathogen(s) of concern detected (5)	–	50
No significant pathogens detected (3)	–	
No facility pathogen history (5)	5	
Facility health capabilities (diagnostics and sampling) (1)		
High (diagnostic and sampling capabilities) (1)	–	5
Medium (sampling capabilities) (3)	–	
Low (require on-site FHC assistance) (5)	5	
Facility type (10)		
Isolation A/quarantine (as defined in 713 FW 1 and 5) (1)	–	70
Isolation B (as defined in 713 FW 1 and 5) (2)	–	
Isolation C (as defined in 713 FW 1 and 5) (3)	–	
Intensive (high environmental control) (5)	–	
Extensive (low environmental control) (7)	7	
Water source (5)		
Closed (protected or enclosed well or spring) (1)	–	25
Open, animal free or treated/disinfected (2)	–	
Open, with any animals (non-treated or non-disinfected) (5)	5	
Cultural impacts on animal health (knowledge of requirements for species) (5)		
Optimal (understand cultural requirements) (1)	–	25
Adequate (incomplete cultural requirements understood) (3)	–	
Unknown (automatically pick "unknown" under facilities) (5)	5	
Cultural impacts on animal health (facilities) (10)		
Optimal (minimal stress for growth, reproduction, or etc.) (1)	–	50
Adequate (for maintenance, potential health problems) (3)	–	
Inadequate (high probability of significant mortalities) (5)		
Unknown (due to "unknown" cultural requirements) (5)	5	
Total risk score		360

Table 5.8 Example completed risk-assessment worksheet for the movement of a hypothetical species, purple sturgeon, from a hypothetical facility. This example represents a low-risk classification

Consideration or factor (factor weight)	Response value	Factor score
Confidence of pathogen surveillance—Methods (5)		
Standard methods (includes lethal) as per Section A of the *Handbook* (1)	1	5
Non-traditional methods (e.g., NWFHS Section C from the *Handbook*) (3)	–	
No surveillance conducted (7)	–	
Confidence of pathogen surveillance—Efforts (5)		
No surveillance conducted (0)	–	5
Standard inspection (includes lethal) to include examination of representative sample of moribund animals (1)	1	
Examination of non-representative sample of animals (4)	–	
Lifestage released (5)		
Gametes/fertilized eggs with parental history of no significant pathogens (1)	–	25
Gametes/fertilized eggs with parental history of significant pathogens (5)	–	
Gametes/fertilized eggs with no parental history (5)	–	
Animal (5)	5	
Pathogen surveillance of proposed propagated population (10)		
High level of population pathogen history (multiple, statistically valid, and lethal samples)		
Significant pathogen(s) detected in population and not known in receiving watershed (5)	–	10
Significant pathogen(s) detected in population and present in receiving watershed (3)	–	
No significant pathogens detected (1)	1	
Low level of population pathogen history (single and/or non-standard samples)	–	Na
Significant pathogen(s) detected in population and not known in receiving watershed (5)	–	
Significant pathogen(s) detected in population and present in receiving watershed (3)	–	
No significant pathogens detected (3)		
No population pathogen history (5)	–	
Receiving watershed (20)		
Same as propagated population's original watershed and facility's watershed (1)	–	20
Same as population's original watershed, not facility's watershed, and closed water supply (1)	1	
Same as population's original watershed, not facility's watershed, and open water supply (3)	–	
Different from population's original watershed and same as facility's (3)	–	
Different from propagated population's original watershed and different from facility's watershed (5)	–	
Total risk score		65

non-inspected 1-month-old juveniles be moved back to the stream of origin (of the original population) for release into the wild.

The resulting health risk score for this situation is 65 (Table 5.8) and equates to a low-risk classification (Table 5.4). The hatchery manager and others involved in the planned move would be informed of the inherent low risk of the movement. A low-risk classification carries with it a recommendation that there be "unrestricted movement out of isolation." In this particular case, the managers would be able to make the planned move to the specified "natal" watershed. If, however, plans were to change to include a different watershed, then the risk would have to be re-evaluated.

Conclusion

The Service's newly revised AAHP and its accompanying reference materials (the *U.S. Fish & Wildlife Service Handbook of Aquatic Animal Health Procedures and Protocols*), is an attempt to proactively maximize the protection of the Nation's natural aquatic resources. The Service is mindful of biosecurity risks associated with movements of aquatic species to and from our NFHs. The AAHP has been revised, in part, to facilitate a documented and uniform animal health risk-assessment of such animal movements, and to provide recommendations relative to the minimization (or elimination) of those risks.

References

USFWS (U.S. Fish & Wildlife Service). 2003a. Risk classification and isolation recommendations for aquatic animals moving onto facilities based on health risk scores. *USFWS Manual*, Part 713, Chapter 5, Exhibit 1. U.S. Fish & Wildlife Service, Washington, DC. On-line version, http://policy.fws.gov/e1713fw5.pdf.

USFWS (U.S. Fish & Wildlife Service). 2003b. Risk classification and isolation recommendations for aquatic animals moving off of facilities based on health risk scores. *USFWS Manual*, Part 713, Chapter 5, Exhibit 2. U.S. Fish & Wildlife Service, Washington, DC. On-line version, http://policy.fws.gov/e2713fw5.pdf.

USFWS (U.S. Fish & Wildlife Service). 2003c. Considerations or factors relative to movements into a facility. *USFWS Form 3-2261*. U.S. Fish & Wildlife Service, Washington, DC. On-line version, http://forms.fws.gov/3-2261.pdf.

USFWS (U.S. Fish & Wildlife Service). 2003d. Considerations or factors relative to movements from a facility.*USFWS Form 3-2262*. U.S. Fish & Wildlife Service, Washington, DC. On-line version, http://forms.fws.gov/3-2262.pdf.

USFWS (U.S. Fish & Wildlife Service). 2004. Isolation level descriptions and definitions. *USFWS Manual*, Part 713, Chapter 5.6, Section F. U.S. Fish & Wildlife Service, Washington, DC. On-line version, http://policy.fws.gov/713fw5.html.

Chapter 6

Wisconsin's Veterinary Approach to Fish Health

Myron J. Kebus

Abstract

Since 1997, the Wisconsin (USA) Department of Agriculture, Trade and Consumer Protection (WDATCP) has developed a regulatory fish health program that creates one set of health standards for both private fish farms and government fish hatcheries. The WDATCP began by working very closely with fish farmers, private veterinary practitioners, and government fish hatchery staff.

The program includes registration of fish farms, certification of veterinarians, rules for health standards for fish introduced into public waters, and issuance of fish import permits. A key component of the Wisconsin fish health program's success has been the close working relationship between WDATCP and fish farmers, and veterinarians.

Introduction

As the Wisconsin markets for farm-raised fish have grown, the need to keep fish healthy on the farm has increased. There are more than 350 commercial fish farms and 1,739 hobby fish farms in Wisconsin. There are also 14 state, two federal, and four tribal hatcheries. The farmers see the investment in fish health as an investment in the future of the $17.5 million aquaculture industry in Wisconsin. The Wisconsin Department of Agriculture, Trade and Consumer Protection (WDATCP) has assisted the Wisconsin aquaculture industry since 1988, initially through the Division of Agricultural Development (previously named the Division of Marketing). In 1997, the Wisconsin Legislature moved the authority for fish health from the Wisconsin Department of Natural Resources (DNR) to WDATCP. With this change, the Division of Animal Health joined the Division of Agricultural Development in 1998 to work together on aquaculture within WDATCP.

E-mail: myron.kebus@datcp.state.wi.us

Wisconsin's fish health program

Beginning in 1997, WDATCP has developed a regulatory fish health program that creates one set of health standards for all private fish farms and government fish hatcheries. Wisconsin law defines fish farms as facilities that hatch or hold fish for the purpose of introduction into the waters of the state, human or animal consumption, recreational fee fishing, and use as bait or fertilizer. In addition to private fish farmers, the WDATCP fish health rules affect Wisconsin DNR hatcheries, DNR cooperative pond growers, tribal hatcheries, University of Wisconsin researchers, high school agriculture classes, and recreational pond owners.

The WDATCP began to develop its fish health program by working very closely with fish farmers, government hatchery staff, and private veterinary practitioners. The WDATCP program includes registration of fish farms, certification of veterinarians, rules for health standards for fish introduced into public waters, and issuance of fish import permits. All farms and facilities must be registered with WDATCP, keep records for 5 years, and make their records available for review by WDATCP Animal Health Inspectors. The records must be kept on fish that were received or delivered.

A key component of the success of the WDATCP program has been the development of fish-farmer friendly and environment friendly solutions to regulatory requirements. For example, health-testing requirements that are affordable and scientifically sound for all fish that are stocked in the state have been developed. In addition, WDATCP has emphasized accurate diagnosis followed by management changes to reduce disease and judicious use of drugs and chemicals. These efforts reduce the risk of unnecessary exposure of farmers, fish, and the environment to harmful substances.

According to a 2001 Wisconsin Legislative Council Information Memorandum (Wisconsin Legislative Council 2001) the WDATCP program has been recognized as a significant accomplishment in the face of declining state budgets. The resources for WDATCP are actually less than most other state fish health programs (WDATCP has the equivalent of only two full-time positions devoted to fish health). In spite of this, according to the UDSA 2002 Census of Agriculture (USDA NASS 2005), Wisconsin ranks third in baitfish production and seventh in trout production in the United States, and has led the United States in efforts to research commercial rearing of yellow perch (*Perca flavescens*).

By training and certifying private practice veterinarians, WDATCP privatized many of the on-farm fish health services that in other states are performed by government employees. This has allowed WDATCP staff to work on progressive efforts, as opposed to working solely on sample collection and submission for disease testing.

The WDATCP Fish Health Program has been very productive. While Wisconsin aquaculture is not as large as that in a number of other states, its representation and influence on national fish health organizations, including the Aquatic Veterinary Medicine Committee of the American Veterinary Medical Association, the National Aquatic Animal Health Task Force, and the U.S. Animal Health Association, have been very strong. Other states, including Ohio, South Dakota, Michigan, and Minnesota, have worked with the WDATCP Fish Health Program to develop regional efforts to strengthen state fish health programs and regulations.

Registration of fish farms

A well-crafted system is now in place that registers all fish farms in the state. As of 15 November 2004, WDATCP had 2,089 registered fish farms. This includes commercial fish farms, state fish hatcheries, and educational fish rearing facilities. Registration aids WDATCP in obtaining critical information (e.g., fish farm locations, species reared, and contact information) that is needed to respond to disease outbreaks. The WDATCP obtains passive surveillance information daily when fish farmers consult the program staff on fish health concerns that include fish morbidity and mortality, water quality, nutrition, and management problems.

The WDATCP maintains a list of reportable fish diseases. "Wisconsin Fish Health Advisories" are widely distributed fish disease fact sheets produced by WDATCP to educate those who raise, transport, and handle farm-raised and wild fish in Wisconsin. The advisories are in a question and answer format that discusses the topics of concern to farmers, such as where diseases have been found, what signs may appear on the fish, and what farmers should do if they suspect a fish disease. The advisories are now used by many other states, and this effort raises the general surveillance of fish diseases in the region. A person who diagnoses or finds evidence of any of the reportable fish diseases is required to report those findings to WDATCP within 10 days.

Record inspection of fish farms is important to validate the registration information. It is followed by compliance efforts that ensure that the fish health rules are being followed equally and fairly throughout the state.

Certification of veterinarians

In the United States and according to Wisconsin state law, veterinarians are "certified" to perform specific specialized veterinary activities, in contrast with "accredited," which denotes the qualification given by the U.S. Department of Agriculture Animal and Plant Health Inspection Service to veterinarians who perform specific functions associated with federal animal health programs. Types of veterinary activities that require certification include certification to perform Johne's disease testing (in cattle), chronic wasting disease testing (in deer), and fish disease testing (in fish).

There was initially a perception by some in the region that fish health would not be adequately served by an agriculture agency and private veterinarians, mostly because it was thought that neither group had sufficient experience with fish. There was no in-state training for WDATCP staff or veterinarians in fish health, so WDATCP developed its own training.

One of the first steps was to hire a program director (Dr. Myron Kebus) in March 1999, who developed and conducted the training for staff, veterinarians, and, subsequently, fish farmers. The WDATCP developed a program to train WDATCP staff and private practice veterinarians on the practical aspects of on-farm water quality and fish medicine procedures and techniques. In April 1999, WDATCP invited all 2,348 of Wisconsin's veterinarians to a series of presentations on Wisconsin aquaculture. The 68 veterinarians who attended the meetings were shown the distribution, size, incomes, and practices of Wisconsin fish farms.

Two months later, WDATCP invited representatives of all registered fish farms (1,725) and the 68 veterinarians who attended the first series of presentations to meet and discuss ideas for linking veterinarians with fish farmers in need of fish health services. A core of 17 veterinarians emerged with a strong interest in providing services to fish farmers. From 1999 to 2002, these veterinarians participated in some of the 13 hands-on, daylong WDATCP veterinary training workshops.

In 2002, the WDATCP fish veterinary training efforts began a collaborative project with the University of Wisconsin–Madison, School of Veterinary Medicine. This led to the development of a new short-course, "Aquaculture Veterinary Medicine for Practitioners," an intensive program designed to provide practical training in field techniques for sample collection and field diagnostics. All veterinarians in Wisconsin who wish to be certified to issue fish health certificates and a "Report of Veterinary Health Assessment of Fish" (Fig. 6.1) must complete the "Aquaculture Veterinary Medicine for Practitioners" course.

The WDATCP also conducted a short course at the South Dakota State University and the Ohio State University in 2004. The collaboration with the University of Wisconsin—Madison, School of Veterinary Medicine has continued with the development of an online version of the course, "Fish Health Medicine Certificate Program," which is due to be available in the autumn of 2005.

Wisconsin has trained and identified more than 75 private veterinary practitioners from nine states, who are certified to issue a "Report of Veterinary Health Assessment of Fish." In addition, the WDATCP maintains a list of aquaculture veterinarians who are accredited by the USDA to perform regulatory services on Wisconsin fish farms.

Health assessment of non-salmonid fish

Fish producers and veterinarians in most states recognize that there are important diseases (e.g., spring viremia of carp [USDA-APHIS 2003], largemouth bass (*Micropterus salmoides*) virus, and heterosporis [WDATCP 2004]) of non-salmonid fish, and that there is a need to develop standards and forms. There are very few examples, in the United States, of health standards and health forms for non-salmonid fish. Thus, many states do not have or are struggling to develop health standards or health forms for non-salmonid fish.

Wisconsin has developed a fish health certificate for all fish introduced to waters of the state and imported to the state. Beginning in 1999, all fish stocked into waters of the state and, in 2001, all fish imported to Wisconsin were required to meet health standards. A valid "Report of Veterinary Health Assessment of Fish" must be provided prior to stocking or importing non-salmonid fish. This Report of Veterinary Health is viewed as a first step in developing health certificates for non-salmonids. Producers have viewed the assessments favorably, largely because they highlight positive findings as well as negative findings, and they are practical, quick, and affordable.

As with many non-salmonid species, there has been very little research on diseases of yellow perch in the United States Common parasitic (*Trichodina* spp., *Gyrodactylus* spp.) and bacterial organisms (*Aeromonas* spp., *Flexibacter* spp.) are seen in Wisconsin yellow perch (Kebus et al. 2004). There have been severe disease outbreaks where a definitive etiology was not determined, including one in 1999 that affected three indoor re-circulating farms simultaneously as a result of importing fish from a farm in Michigan. The brain parasite *Myxobolus neurophilus* has not been reported in Wisconsin, but remains a significant concern (Acland et al. 2002). The muscle parasite *Heterosporis* sp. has been reported in lakes and streams in Wisconsin, but not in fish farms. Digenean flukes are very common and

Date of Inspection: __________ Prior Inspection Dates: __________ __________ __________

Name of Fish Source	Address or Location of Fish Source	Name of Owner or Manager	Fish Farm Registration #

Type of Water Supply (check all that apply): ___ Spring ___ Stream ___ Well ___ UV Treated ___ Lake or Impoundment ___ Enclosed ___ Free of Fish

NOTE: A minimum of 20 fish of each species must be examined					PARAMETERS ASSESSED FOR Numbers Sampled (Line 1) and Results (Line 2)										
Species[1]	Lot Number	Age[2]	Number in Lot	Obtained as Eggs (E) or Fish (F) from	AV LN	AV WT	Eyes	Skin	Fins	Gills	Liver	Kidney	Spleen	Fat	Muscle

Remarks
Drug and Chemical History:
Skin Scrap:
Gill Mount:

Name, Address, Telephone Number and License Number of Fish Health Veterinarian or Fish Health Inspector

Signature of Fish Health Veterinarian or Fish Health Inspector:
In my professional opinion I did not see any significant sign of contagious or infectious disease.

[1] Use standard abbreviations (see below)
[2] For hatchery fish, give the age in months; for feral fish, use one of the following: E-eggs or fry F-fingerlings Y-yearlings B-older fish

File copy with: Wisconsin Department of Agriculture, Trade & Consumer Protection
Division of Animal Health
P.O. Box 8911, Madison, WI 53708-8911
Telephone: 608-224-4872 Fax: 608-224-4871

Fig. 6.1 Report of Veterinary Health Assessment of Fish, developed by the Wisconsin Department of Agriculture, Trade & Consumer Protection (WDATCP) (*Continues*).

Standard Species Abbreviations

AMP	Amur pike	FRD	Freshwater drum	OTP	Other pike
ARG	Arctic grayling	GAR	Gar	OTS	Other sucker
ATS	Atlantic salmon	GIT	Gila trout	PAH	Paddlefish
BCF	Blue catfish	GOF	Goldfish	PKS	Pink salmon
BCFCCF	Blue catfish x channel catfish	GOS	Golden shiner	RBT	Rainbow trout
BIB	Bigmouth buffalo	GOT	Golden trout	RBTSTT	Rainbow trout x steelhead trout
BKT	Brook trout	GRC	Grass carp	RSF	Redear sunfish
BLB	Black bullhead	GSF	Green sunfish	SAB	Smallmouth buffalo
BLC	Black crappie	HEG	Herring	SAR	Sauger
BLG	Bluegill	KIH	Killifish	SCS	Spring chinook salmon
BLGHYB	Hybrid bluegill	KOE	Kokanee	SMB	Smallmouth bass
BLP	Blue pike	LAS	Landlocked Atlantic salmon	SOS	Sockeye salmon
BNT	Brown trout	LAT	Lake trout	SPB	Spotted bass
BON	Bowfin	LAY	Lamprey	STB	Striped bass
BRB	Brown bullhead	LIR	Livebearer	STK	Stickleback
CAP	Carp	LMB	Largemouth bass	STN	Sturgeon
CCF	Channel catfish	MOE	Mooneye	STT	Steelhead trout
CHS	Chum salmon	MCS	Miscellaneous warm water	SVC	Silver carp
COS	Coho salmon	MUE	Muskellunge	WAE	Walleye
CUT	Cutthroat trout	MUW	Mudminnow	WAESAR	Walleye x sauger
DAR	Darters	NOP	Northern pike	WAM	Warmouth
DOV	Dolly varden	OCF	Other catfish	WCF	White catfish
DOVBKT	Dolly varden x brook trout	OHT	Ohrid trout	WCS	Winter chinook salmon
FCF	Flathead catfish	OSA	Other salmonid	WSK	White sucker
FCS	Fall chinook salmon	OSF	Other sunfish	YPC	Yellow perch
FHM	Fathead minnow	OTM	Other minnow	. . .	. . .

Fig. 6.1 (*Continued*).

affect fillet quality of pond-reared yellow perch. They can render fillets unacceptable for consumers, yet their impact on fish health remains unclear.

In spite of economic losses due to yellow perch diseases, the discussion of yellow perch health has been generally secondary to issues of feed training, rearing, nutrition, and marketing. Producers often realize the importance of the disease late in the process of learning to rear yellow perch. The most severe yellow perch health problems have been observed in re-circulating tank systems. Water quality problems have been a major contributing factor in these health problems. There are significant health concerns with pond rearing, though to-date reports of fish health problems in ponds have been fewer than reports from re-circulating tank systems.

The "Report of Veterinary Health Assessment of Fish" conducted on yellow perch has strengthened Wisconsin's general surveillance of yellow perch diseases, which have limited production and contributed to the failure of a dozen major farms. These farms, which have invested an estimated cumulative $16 million in the upper Midwest, including Wisconsin, are an economically important sector of aquaculture in the region.

Fish import permits

Fish are transported into Wisconsin from 26 states and Canada. In 2003, Wisconsin imported 726 metric tons (1.6 million lbs) of fathead minnows (*Pimephales promelas*), 202 metric tons (445,000 lbs) of golden shiners (*Notemigonus crysoleucas*), 272 metric tons (600,000 lbs) of white sucker (*Catostomus commersoni*), 374,000 walleye (*Stizostedion vitreum*), and 6 million yellow perch.

A person importing live fish or fish eggs into Wisconsin must first obtain an annual import permit from WDATCP. The import permit is issued only when a valid Report of Veterinary Health Assessment has been approved by WDATCP. Then, the import permit is issued to the Wisconsin facility that will receive the imported fish. They send or fax a copy of the permit to those who will deliver the fish from out of the state. The hauler is required to carry a copy of the permit during transport.

Since 1997, WDATCP has issued over 750 import permits for fish originating from 26 states and from Canada. In 2003, 105 fish import permits were issued, which is similar to the number issued in 2001 and 2002.

Conclusion

While WDATCP has made substantial progress in developing fish health standards that apply to everyone, there are numerous challenges ahead. A key reason for the success of WDATCP has been the development of regulations that balance a broad range of shareholder's concerns and fish health concerns.

One of the challenges will be to characterize the economic impact of diseases of various fish health problems. If successful, this could advance the progress of the WDATCP fish health program, since the more that standards and rules are shown to increase profitability, the more they will be adopted and supported.

With some species of fish, very little is known about the disease organisms and their impact on health. The WDATCP program will benefit from more sound scientific information on disease organisms and their importance in fish diseases. The standards and rules will need to be modified to reflect the emerging knowledge of disease organisms and health.

In the future, the WDATCP fish health program may develop science-based best management standards for farm-raised fish, increase fish health standards, and refine current understanding of the relationships between fish health, food safety, and environmental stewardship.

Leadership will also involve the coordination of the various stakeholders within the state such as fish farmers, pond owners, private veterinary practitioners, other state agencies, universities, diagnostic labs, and tribes. Communication among these stakeholders will be critical in the development of the aquaculture industry.

While the North Central states share similar aquatic environmental conditions and even watersheds, fish health regulations vary tremendously from state to state. Wisconsin has worked with other states to characterize the patchwork of fish health regulations and works toward regional harmonization of fish health regulations. Fish health regulatory issues have been contentious, and "trade barriers" have been established under the guise of fish health protection. The harmonization of interstate fish health regulations will be a major factor in determining the fate of aquaculture development in the region.

Acknowledgments

The author expresses sincere thanks to Dr. Robert Ehlenfeldt, Will Hughes, Gin Gronli, and Donna Gilson for their efforts in the development of the WDATCP fish health program.

References

Acland, H., H. Rodger, and F. Rommel. 2002. Brain parasite in cultured yellow perch (abstract). *In 25th Annual Eastern Fish Health Workshop*. Kearneysville, WV, 10–13 March 2000. U.S. Geological Survey Leetown Science Center, Kearneysville, WV. On-line, http://www.lsc.usgs.gov/FHB/workshops/25/39.htm.

Kebus, M.J., T.P. Barry, and J.A. Malison, editors. 2004. *Percis III. Proceedings of the Third International Percid Fish Symposium*. Madison, WI, 20–24 July 2003. University of Wisconsin Sea Grant, Madison, WI. 136 pp.

USDA–APHIS (United States Department of Agriculture, Animal and Plant Health Inspection Services). 2003. *APHIS Factsheet*. Spring viremia of carp. On-line, http://www.aphis.usda.gov/lpa/pubs/fsheet_faq_notice/fs_ahcarp.pdf.

USDA NASS (United States Department of Agriculture, National Agricultural Statistics Service). 2005. *2002 Census of Agriculture*. USDA NASS, Washington, DC. On-line, http://www.nass.usda.gov/census/census02/volume1/USVolume104.pdf.

WDATCP (Wisconsin Department of Agriculture, Trade & Consumer Protection). 2004. *Fish Health*. On-line version, http://www.datcp.state.wi.us/ah/agriculture/animals/aqua/health.

Wisconsin Legislative Council. 2001. *Wisconsin Legislative Council Information Memorandum. Aquaculture: A Maturing Agricultural Sector*, http://www.legis.state.wi.us/lc.

Chapter 7

Harmonized, Standardized, and Flexible National Frameworks for Ensuring Diagnostic Data and Test Result Validity: A Critical Need for Aquatic Animal Health Diagnostic Systems and for Biosecurity in Aquaculture

Ann L. Wiegers, Jerry R. Heidel, and A. David Scarfe

Abstract

Valid data and test results are critical for the control and eradication of aquatic animal diseases and pathogens. Valid data and test results are also important to biosecurity-related activities, including health certification, surveillance and monitoring programs, epidemiological studies, recognition of emerging diseases, and rapid, effective response to animal health emergencies.

For analytical and diagnostic validity, laboratory competence to conduct testing and related activities must be verified. Demonstration of competence is achieved with appropriate documented policies, systems, procedures, and scientifically sound specifications that meet the requirements of third-party consensus standards. Verification of meeting requirements is obtained by nationally and internationally recognized third-party laboratory accreditation.

There are four areas of competence regarding valid data and test results: the conduct of testing, the use of valid test methods, proficiency testing, and the use of reference materials. This chapter reviews the standards used in each of these four areas. The bases for requirements for laboratory accreditation, accreditation body recognition programs, and the organizations that support these programs are examined. These elements have been discussed previously (Wiegers et al. 2003, 2004). The chapter explains how a harmonized national system of accreditation, meeting applicable international standards, may assist in creating a sound national laboratory system. It also explains how

---

Ann L. Wiegers, corresponding author. E-mail: Ann.L.Wiegers@aphis.usda.gov

one may effectively address the need for data and test result validity, credibility, standardization, and harmonization while allowing the flexibility necessary to create a robust national system that can effectively deliver reliable diagnostic testing and respond to contingency planning. Direct application of the presented concepts is illustrated and related to the current organization of aquatic animal health diagnostic testing in the United States.

Introduction

The rapid, accurate diagnosis of aquatic animal disease is becoming increasingly important to aquatic and wild aquatic animal populations, particularly in commercial trade and environmental replenishment. There is increasing concern regarding World Organisation for Animal Health (OIE) notifiable and other important diseases that are endemic in many areas and regarding outbreaks of introduced aquatic animal disease. Biosecurity is now a priority for all aquatic animal industries, and the focal point is diagnosing disease or infection.

The number of laboratories and individuals performing aquatic animal disease diagnosis, and available diagnostic tests for aquatic animals are increasing rapidly. Valid data and test results are essential for verifying health status, identifying disease, and epidemiological efforts. Data and test results are under increased scrutiny in programs that require disease prevention, control, and eradication. Laboratories are under mounting pressure to provide assurance to their clients and stakeholders, that their testing services are accurate and that their facilities meet the standards expected by trading partners. Clients, the end users of results, include those wanting to know the health (or disease) status of animals under their care, those receiving animals or animal products, and state, federal, and international regulators working to prevent the introduction of disease. The need for increased reliance on data and test results indicates that aquatic animal industries and health specialists must examine the elements and processes underlying the production of data and test results.

This chapter discusses national and international requirements for laboratory standards, laboratory accreditation, and accreditation bodies recognized in the United States and internationally. Four critical areas of competency are discussed: the conduct of testing, the use of valid test methods, proficiency testing, and the use of reference materials. Recent U.S. legislation and resulting standards and activities have established a unified national system of accreditation that meets applicable international standards. This is also discussed. In addition, this chapter discusses how data and test result validity, credibility, standardization, and harmonization can be achieved while allowing the flexibility needed to create a strong and responsive national diagnostic system. This information is related to the current organizational situation regarding aquatic animal health diagnostic tests and diagnostic laboratories in the United States.

Elements of laboratory systems

A national laboratory system that can provide reliable diagnostic services necessary for biosecurity, and rapid and effective responses to animal health emergencies must have:

- well-characterized, reliable reference materials of sufficient shelf life, quantity, and availability, for use in test development, validation, and comparison;

- valid, well-controlled, and well-documented test methods;
- official guidance on test result application and interpretation;
- an effective method evaluation and approval process;
- a valid and effective method transfer process (e.g., verifying that the method is in statistical control at the user site, formal analyst training, verification of successful training, and training for the "field," or sample submitters, to ensure that the samples are fit to use on arrival);
- valid processes to determine analyst and laboratory proficiency to perform the test (i.e., valid proficiency test materials and programs);
- valid processes to compare different test methods; and
- valid processes to compare the same method in different laboratories or among analysts.

The items above have usually been supplied by reference laboratories, typically those at which the recognized technical expertise resides (e.g., a national, most frequently federal laboratory or an OIE reference laboratory). In a national emergency, reference laboratories may have to rely on test results, materials, or data from other laboratories. These others may be asked to use reference laboratory validated, evaluated, and approved test methods in a national emergency or for federal programs (e.g., National Animal Health Laboratory Network (NAHLN) laboratories, contract laboratories, federally approved laboratories). A national laboratory system must therefore have

- flexibility within a framework of consistency;
- the ability to respond quickly and to handle a sudden large increase in samples to be tested ("surge capacity," or a constant state of "readiness to perform" specific testing);
- the ability to compare test results;
- *demonstrated competence* in data gathering (i.e., research and development), in conducting routine and non-routine testing, in reference material characterization and production, in method development, validation, evaluation, and transfer, and in the conduct of proficiency testing, as applicable;
- dispassionate, consistent, and expert verification of competence: a valid third-party laboratory recognition (approval or accreditation) system; and
- international recognition of competence.

Those charged with the creation and maintenance of an effective national biosecurity system have concerns regarding the demonstration of due diligence in decisions concerning the acceptance of test results. These include who will be allowed to determine test method performance, deliver expert interpretation or diagnosis, or confirm diagnoses; how methods used in a national emergency or in national surveillance programs will be validated and approved; who will be allowed to do testing; and how these decisions will be justified to the public and trading partners.

The national system must be flexible, prepared to make the best use of the best technical expertise, wherever that may reside, and be able to allocate or reallocate resources. The national system must be quickly expandable in the diagnostic area of need.

These resources, tasks, and processes *all rest on the foundation of competence to produce valid data and test results and to interpret them*, and encompass valid methods, proficiency testing, and reference materials. Consistency is acquired by the use of general standards that may be used to *recognize competence* in these areas.

Trading partners must be assured that the national system is effective in disease diagnosis, surveillance, and control. Thus, there is a need to speak in a common "currency" in the recognition of competence that requires harmonization by the use of national and international standards in the recognition of competence.

Regulators have relied on a type of third-party competence verification known as laboratory (or analyst) *approval. Approvals* are administered by the regulatory authority to determine who may do testing work and rely largely on federal resident technical expertise, and federal training and oversight. Highly pragmatic, and generally technical and task oriented, approval can be effective, but is not consistent over all of government or from test method to test method, as it is program- or disease-oriented. The same test method may be used differently from laboratory to laboratory, depending on the needs and priorities. In some instances, the approved laboratory may choose any one component or all of any licensed test kit. This can make comparison of results difficult. A great deal of resources and expertise are required to administer federal approval programs. In times of need and national crisis, approval can be cumbersome. Accreditation bodies could be used to assist in approval, but these bodies did not or do not necessarily conduct their work according to accepted national or international standards. Neither were nor are these bodies necessarily assessed for competence to award accreditations. Trading partners may well ask, "Who is guarding the guardians?"

International and national accreditation systems, including those developed in and endorsed by the United States, have been developed. These systems rely on the use of international standards produced by reputable international standards organizations. In the United States, their use is supported by legislation. The United States also has obligations to conform to the requirements of these standards, as outlined by law, treaty, or other mutual agreements (Wiegers 2002).

Demonstration of competence

Data and test result validity are defined in part by recent legislation. The National Technology Transfer and Advancement Act (NTTAA) of 1996 set the stage in the United States for the use of third-party, internationally accepted consensus standards and laboratory accreditation in lieu of regulatory activity and in support of trade. The U.S. Congress assigned to the National Institute of Standards and Technology (NIST), Department of Commerce, the responsibility to coordinate and set standards for laboratory accreditation activities of Federal, State, and local entities with those of the private sector. The NIST was also assigned the responsibility to eliminate unnecessary duplication and complexity in the development and promulgation of such measures, and to provide harmonization with international standards. To these ends, NIST helped to establish the National Cooperation for Laboratory Accreditation (NACLA) in 1998. The NACLA recognizes accreditation bodies and conducts its work using guides and standards endorsed by the International Cooperation for Laboratory Accreditation (ILAC). The ILAC, which is the established standards maker for laboratory accreditation internationally, relies heavily on third-party consensus standards, including those of the International Organization for Standardization (ISO) and the International

Electrotechnical Commission (IEC). The ISO is probably the foremost standards writing body in the world, and produces standards using large, international committees composed of technical experts according to a rigorous, established process. These standards are internationally recognized, and U.S. endorsement of their use for laboratory accreditation has been an important step forward in ensuring test results are valid and in ensuring that test results produced in the United States are accepted internationally. A more detailed discussion of laboratory accreditation in the United States and internationally can be found elsewhere (Wiegers 2002).

Legislation, international standards bodies, and therefore U.S. accreditation bodies have thus defined what the expectations of users of laboratory data and test results should be. They have created a sound foundation and framework within which to build national laboratory systems. Expectations center on the demonstration of competence in four areas of key importance: (a) to conduct testing, (b) to develop, validate, and approve test methods for use, (c) to operate proficiency testing programs, and (d) to produce and distribute reference materials.

Currently, laboratory responsibilities in aquatic animal health testing are shared by federal, state, academic, tribal, and private laboratories. Guidance regarding recommended practices for aquatic animal testing has been provided by organizations such as the OIE (2002, 2003), the Fish Health Section of the American Fisheries Society (AFS-FHS), and the U.S. Department of Agriculture, Animal and Plant Health Inspection Service (USDA-APHIS). Functional roles, responsibilities, jurisdictions, and inter-relationships, however, while at least partly defined, are often not well understood or particularly clear. The diversity of aquatic animal health laboratories makes establishing a uniform system of laboratory quality management and test validation and approval an extremely complex task. Until recently, a solid, internationally compatible national laboratory recognition framework has not been in place to establish general required practices or to support data and test result validity and credibility. The adoption and use of internationally accepted guidance and standards for laboratory and accreditation body recognition in critical diagnostic or testing areas, including those offered by the OIE and ILAC, have now made the creation of a credible, efficient, effective, and synergistic national aquatic animal health laboratory network more easily attainable. The use of the ILAC and NACLA endorsed standards does not conflict with the use of OIE standards (specified in treaty and trade agreements), i.e., OIE requirements must be met or exceeded, and there is no obligation to use the actual document. The OIE standards may be incorporated into NACLA requirements as necessary.

Testing, validation of methods, proficiency testing, and reference materials are not standalone measures. Each is dependent on the other to ensure a reliable result. Each, however, is discussed separately in this chapter, to cover the standards and accreditations available.

Competence is demonstrated by third-party accreditation

The ISO/IEC Guide 2 defines accreditation as "a procedure by which an authoritative body gives formal recognition that a body or person is competent to carry out specific tasks" (ISO 2004a). The use of the term "certification" is not equivalent to accreditation and does not imply competence (e.g., certification or registration of a quality system to ISO 9001

(ISO 2000c). "Laboratory accreditation" is the formal recognition of the competence of a laboratory to carry out specific tests or specific types of tests (ISO 2004a).

Accreditation to produce test results

As mentioned, in the United States, NACLA recognizes the authoritative bodies that accredit laboratories according to ILAC requirements. In the United States and internationally, competence to conduct testing is defined by the requirements of ISO/IEC 17025, *General requirements for the competence of testing and calibration laboratories* (ISO 2005), the standard required by ILAC. This standard is comprehensive, detailed, and has both quality system and technical requirements. It is a general standard, and precisely how to implement the technical and managerial requirements is left to the laboratory. This is one of its strengths, as it can be adapted to any particular scientific or diagnostic discipline or any program. Requirements include adequate facilities, accurate equipment, qualified staff, appropriately validated test methods, and a comprehensive and effective quality management system. Testing and calibration laboratories that comply with ISO/IEC 17025 are considered to also operate in accordance with the ISO 9000 standards (ISO 2000b, 2000c, 2000d), normative references. ISO/IEC 17025 also forms the basis for OIE requirements for veterinary diagnostic testing (OIE 2002, 2003), for both terrestrial and aquatic animals. This concordance is significant, as it unites U.S. legislative requirements (i.e., the NTTAA) with trade arrangements under which the United States must meet or exceed OIE requirements. Clauses in ISO/IEC 17025 concerning subcontracting and method validation support the need for the use of ISO/IEC 17025 in all laboratories involved in a national laboratory system or network, particularly if different laboratories are to do screening and confirmatory testing, and if test validation and the production of proficiency samples and reference materials are done by laboratories other than the user laboratories.

Accreditation bodies will accredit private, government, industry, or academic laboratories and will also create special accreditation programs in specialized areas, such as food microbiology. The choice of an accreditation body is especially important if the accreditation is to be recognized for commerce or regulatory control. The ILAC and therefore NACLA require that accreditation bodies using ISO/IEC 17025 meet the requirements of ISO/IEC 17011 (ISO 2004b). These are intended to ensure the competence of the accreditation body to accredit a laboratory, include requirements for the organization of the accreditation body, for its quality system, for how the accreditation body grants, maintains, extends, suspends, and withdraws accreditation, for its documentation, for its requirements for laboratory assessors and for how the assessors are qualified and contracted, and for how the accreditation process is handled (from application to granting accreditation, and including surveillance and reassessment).

Recognition by NACLA of the accreditation body completes the testing recognition package, and NACLA has already recognized many, directly or by a memorandum of understanding, including those capable of accrediting veterinary laboratories.

Accreditation for testing may bring several other benefits besides recognition and acceptance of competence. These include increased productivity, improved performance, improved efficiency, increased staff morale, credentials to qualify for testing work, ability to compete in some markets, an objective assessment, opportunities for improvement, increased opportunity to stay current of developments in requirements for competence and testing, and possible decreases in the cost of liability insurance. The users of the laboratory results obtain confidence in the results and therefore greater confidence in the appropriateness of their application.

Accreditation has associated costs. These include costs for implementation and maintenance of requirements and for the accreditation. These will vary and are beyond the scope of this chapter to discuss in detail. Major factors affecting the cost of accreditation include the size of the laboratory, the location of the laboratory, the scope, type, and field(s) of testing desired to be on the certificate of accreditation, the gap between the status of the laboratory and the requirements for accreditation, and the fees required by the selected accreditation body. Information on fees may be obtained from each accreditation body. Each laboratory, having approximated the cost of accreditation, should also carefully consider the cost of not having the accreditation. Also, the international situation is such that accreditation should be considered as the cost of doing certain types of testing business.

Accreditation of other key areas

Regarding accreditation for the following areas of endeavor, as test results are generated in support of these activities, a laboratory seeking accreditation in these areas should first have an accreditation to ISO/IEC 17025, since competence to conduct method validation, proficiency testing, and reference material production and distribution is dependant on the competence to conduct testing.

Method validation

Accreditation alone will not necessarily yield a valid test result if the test methods used have not been properly validated or have been poorly chosen. Validation is defined as "confirmation by examination and the provision of objective evidence that the particular requirements for a specific intended use are fulfilled" (ISO 2004a). Reputable, approved sources of valid methods are essential for a laboratory system. Although ISO/IEC 17025 does not specify the methods to be used, there are requirements for method validation. Some NACLA recognized accreditation bodies accredit laboratories for competence to conduct test development and validation. Non-routine testing may be viewed as a type of method development and validation (CITAC 1998). Because non-routine testing is the rule for many real or potential emergencies, competence in this area is critical.

Common strategic errors in the choice and implementation of test methods are to focus on the technical aspects of validation alone, and to overemphasize the importance of numbers of samples or test results used in the validation. Attention must be paid to the management of the method validation and method approval processes. It is essential to obtain the informed approval of the client (user of the test method and test results) regarding method performance characteristics and risks involved. For example, the level of confidence in calculated performance characteristics such as diagnostic and analytical cutoff, sensitivity, and specificity is dependent on the number of samples tested in the method validation. Factors such as costs, deadlines, and availability of materials may lower the sample numbers, lowering confidence in the accuracy and precision of these calculated characteristics. The client, however, may agree to a lower confidence if costs are high and the deadline is short, especially if the impact of a wrong answer is relatively light. Client approval is particularly important if the client is a jurisdictional authority authorizing use of official methods or the allowance of specific tolerances. The method approval process, as well as the client and stakeholder involvement in selection, development, validation, approval, and transfer, is critical to ensure that the best method for the intended purpose is used. The processes by which a method is selected, developed, evaluated, approved for use, transferred, and further evaluated for fitness for a particular situation may be equally important or more important than the amount of data used to support the performance characteristics of the method. As one generates test results while developing and evaluating methods, it is highly desirable that the validating laboratory have an accreditation to ISO/IEC 17025, and that the method development and validation data have been produced in a quality management system as specified therein. The necessary characteristics of a valid method have been listed and discussed (Wiegers 2003).

Imported methods should be selected from reputable sources (e.g., the AOAC International, formerly the Association of Official Analytical Chemists), or be further validated or evaluated by the testing laboratory. Methods used for the calibration of testing equipment must also be valid.

Many reputable technical organizations provide guidance on various aspects of method validation and approval. These include the AOAC International, the Cooperation on International Traceability in Analytical Chemistry, the International Union of Pure and Applied Chemistry, the American Society for Testing and Materials, the National Committee for Clinical Laboratory Standards, and the OIE. The AOAC International has a well-established, very well-respected method validation program. The U.S. Food and Drug Administration, the U.S. Department of Agriculture, and other state and federal agencies use the validated, published methods of AOAC International. They are cited in regulations. Documented test methods having gone through an endorsed and established validation and approval process are sometimes known as "official methods." The use of the term "standard methods" is confusing unless specifically defined in the text (see OIE 2003), and the quality of the methods endorsed by the official method process rests on the content and requirements of that process. The AOAC International endorses ISO/IEC 17025, and its method validation process meets ISO/IEC requirements in this area.

Proficiency testing

Proficiency testing is needed to ensure that analysts and laboratories may successfully use a valid documented method. Proficiency testing is also critical in comparing results between laboratories using the same method (identifying differences) and to compare or monitor methods. Proficiency testing may also be used to determine performance characteristics of a method in a collaborative trial, to assign values to reference materials, or to determine their suitability for use. In some cases, proficiency tested samples may also be considered as reference materials.

Participation in proficiency testing is a strong guideline of ISO/IEC 17025, and is a requirement for accreditation in the United States. Such programs are now considered to be an integral part of a national laboratory system. For a client or a user laboratory to have confidence in a proficiency testing program, it is necessary that proficiency test materials and panel members ("samples") be properly chosen, prepared, characterized, preserved, labeled, and distributed. A system of true blinding (e.g., coding or otherwise preparing the "samples" to ensure that the answers are unknown to the analyst) must be devised and appropriately applied. "Pass/fail" and other comparative criteria must be established in a statistically valid way, and correctly applied. Confidentiality must be ensured. Proficiency testing is critical to the acceptance of test results for trade and regulatory purposes, and ISO, ILAC, and accreditation bodies have produced comprehensive general guidance for the accreditation of proficiency testing providers (ISO 1997a, 1997b; ILAC 2000b). Accreditation is available. Requirements include

- a quality management system for the proficiency testing program;
- staff (technicians, technical experts) and collaborators (subcontracted laboratories) with the necessary technical, statistical, and administrative expertise, and with the necessary authority and resources;
- a program coordinator, technical manager, and quality manager;
- a program plan;
- data processing equipment;
- documented and valid statistical models and data analysis techniques;
- procedures for coordination and operation of the program;
- instructions for the proficiency testing participants (e.g., handling, testing, reporting results); and
- policy and procedures for test material and test item preparation, management, and storage; homogeneity and stability testing, packaging, labeling, and distribution; data analysis and interpretation, records, program reports, evaluation of performance, communication with participants, document control, contract review, procurement, client feedback, control of non-conforming work, internal audit, corrective and preventive action, management review, and confidentiality and ethical considerations.

The AOAC International proficiency testing program is accredited by the American Association for Laboratory Accreditation (A2LA), a NACLA recognized accreditation body. As the production of proficiency-tested samples requires testing, it would be desirable for collaborator laboratories to be accredited to ISO/IEC 17025. A more detailed discussion of proficiency testing may be found elsewhere (Wiegers 2004).

Reference material production and distribution

Reference materials are a type of reference standard and may be defined as materials that have components, properties, or values that are sufficiently well-established or characterized by repetitive, expert analysis or measurement under specialized, controlled conditions to the extent that they may be used as or in the establishment of a "true" or accepted value (e.g., an American Type Culture Collection organism or a positive antiserum from a national reference laboratory). A reference material will therefore also have properties that render it suitable to be used for equipment calibration, method validation, or the establishment of controls for a test method (e.g., positive and negative antisera). The use of the term "standard reference material" can be misleading. It is preferable to indicate whether a particular reference material is used as a technical or measurement standard (e.g., in testing animal biologics, as a "reference standard"). Reference materials are critical in ensuring that data, test results, laboratories, and test methods may be compared in an objective, controlled manner. They are critical in test method development and design. As such, apart from valid data and test results, reference materials provide the most important component of test validation and control and may be used in, as well as created by, proficiency testing programs. As they can create a normative basis for communications about method performance and the interpretation or applicability of test results, they are the most important validity topic discussed in this chapter, and it is essential to the credibility of a national testing system that the producers of reference materials be able to demonstrate competence in conducting their production and validation.

Accreditation for reference material production is or will soon be available by recognized accreditation bodies. The ILAC has produced the guidance that forms the basis for the accreditation of reference materials producers (ILAC 2000a). The ILAC guidelines are largely based on the requirements of ISO Guide 34 (ISO 2000a). The production of reference materials involves the production of test results, so the requirements of ISO/IEC 17025 apply.

ISO Guide 34 describes requirements for the competence of reference material producers and is intended to be used for their accreditation. These general requirements are complex, comprehensive, and include the following.

- Management system requirements that include a quality management system;
- Requirements for document control, contract review, use of collaborators (subcontractors), procurement, dealing with client feedback, control of non-conforming work (reference materials), records, internal audit, corrective and preventive action, and management review; and
- Technical requirements for management, staffing, and training at the producer's laboratory, collaborators, production planning, production control, the production environment, material preparation, assessment of homogeneity and stability, measurement methods and equipment, traceability, characterization, assignment of values and their uncertainties, certificates and supporting information, handling and storage, packing, labeling, dispatch, records, reports, and post-distribution service.

Conclusion

The United States has implemented a laboratory accreditation system to meet critical national needs. This new system can help ensure that a sound, responsive national laboratory system is available and will meet international requirements. Recognition based on *competence* promotes consistency within a framework of requirements. The ability to accredit pieces of the system (e.g., testing, proficiency testing, reference material production) supports efforts such as the National Animal Health Emergency Monitoring System and the NAHLN, allowing the fullest possible participation by non-federal laboratories, reducing replication of effort, enhancing effective communication, and establishing and maintaining validity and credibility. It supports international acceptance of test results and data.

The required standards are complementary. This helps to implement requirements with minimal effort, and ISO/IEC 17025 quality system requirements implemented in one area will more easily enable implementation of quality system requirements in other critical areas. For example, if a document control system is already implemented for testing, one can add the additional documents required for proficiency testing and reference materials to the extant system. The use of national and international standards also provides a "common currency" and vocabulary of communication, facilitating efficient and effective collaboration.

The technical requirements of ISO/IEC 17025 promote and support good scientific principles and practices. If technical requirements are embedded in a quality management system based on international standards and recognized third-party accreditation, then industry and national security will reap significant benefits, including improvement in trade position, enhanced animal health, better protection from litigation, and an effective response during animal health emergencies.

The requirements of the discussed ISO/IEC standards are comprehensive, yet general. This ensures that testing laboratories, test developers, proficiency test providers, and reference material producers can interpret and implement the requirements according to the testing services provided, technical requirements, standards established by technical experts, or client and stakeholder needs. The standards say "what," but not "how," allowing the flexibility to make adjustments, and ensuring that accreditation standards can be interpreted for varied federal or public programs for specific testing areas. Technical specifications or administrative policy need not be superseded.

The reputation of a laboratory, the credibility of a regulatory program, the satisfaction of clients, the public safety, and the health and well-being of countless animals depend on reliable test methods, valid and timely laboratory results, well-characterized and stable proficiency testing materials, well-designed and executed proficiency testing programs, and a dependable supply of reliable reference materials. These contribute to a sound technical base for producing, interpreting, and reporting reliable test results, and verify that users can conduct the valid test method in a manner that yields reliable results.

Public and private laboratories devoted to the diagnosis of diseases of aquatic animals are found throughout the United States. These include those supporting state, academic, federal, and tribal agencies and institutions. At this time, there is no single, unified, or common system of laboratory accreditation for aquatic animal health laboratories. State supported, full service veterinary laboratories, located in state departments of agriculture or colleges of veterinary medicine, provide services for all animal species and may have sections devoted to aquatics. Some may adhere to standards used in laboratory accreditation by the American Association of Veterinary Laboratory Diagnosticians (AAVLD). Due to the limitations imposed by the AAVLD, however, only state laboratories can currently participate, and the AAVLD is not NACLA recognized. The USDA–APHIS provides an "approval" for public and private laboratories providing fish health certification for international trade.

The subsequent lack of consistency in standards among aquatic laboratories carries with it the obvious potential for variability. This can be viewed as a weakness by stakeholders, including the public and international trading partners, and could negatively impact user confidence and commerce.

Thus, it is important that laboratory standards meeting international standards be implemented in aquatic animal health laboratories. In this way, the United States will be able to quickly and consistently identify and respond to health emergencies with informed decisions based on reliable data. The NACLA system of accreditation is ready to assist in ensuring that these goals are met. Under NACLA, it is hoped that regulators will "recognize" a laboratory accredited by a NACLA-recognized accreditation body (i.e., meeting the requirements of ISO/IEC 17025) as meeting federal approval requirements.

Preferably, however, approval programs will be replaced with the NACLA system of accreditation.

Accreditation bodies recognized by NACLA can and will create special programs, based on ISO/IEC 17025, for specific test or diagnostic areas. In these programs, specific technical requirements are added. For example, in the A2LA special accreditation program for food testing, additional technical requirements are added to the basic ISO/IEC 17025 requirements (A2LA 2002). Accreditation bodies have also partnered with regulators in verifying specific contractual obligations of laboratories contracted or approved to do federal testing work. For example, the accreditation body can verify that only approved or official methods are used, and that other specified technical and procedural requirements are met. Accredited proficiency test providers can partner with government to administer proficiency testing programs. For example, proficiency test materials and panels can be created at laboratories where the technical expertise resides, but the program can be administered by the accredited provider. The flexibility built into these systems makes many options possible, and can save government resources. Through accreditation, aquatic animal health laboratories can fulfill their service role to the aquaculture industry, natural resource agencies, and the public. All laboratory clients, whether they are countries, governmental agencies, large corporations, small businesses, or individuals, will feel confident that test results are valid.

Acknowledgments

Thanks to Drs. Louise Henderson, Michel Carr, David Dusek, Melisse Schilling, and Linda Schlater of the Center for Veterinary Biologics; and Dr. Beverly Schmitt of the National Veterinary Services Laboratories for comments on the manuscript.

References

A2LA (The American Association for Laboratory Accreditation). 2002. *A2LA Food Testing Program Requirements*. The American Association for Laboratory Accreditation, Frederick, MD. 1 p.

CITAC (Cooperation on International Traceability in Analytical Chemistry). 1998. *Eurachem/CITAC Guide CG 2. Quality Assurance for Research and Development and Non-routine Analysis*. The CITAC Secretariat, IRMM, Retieseweg, Belgium. 67 pp.

ILAC (The International Laboratory Accreditation Cooperation). 2000a. *ILAC-G12: Guidelines for the Requirements for the Competence of Reference Material Producers*. ILAC Secretariat, Rhodes, New South Wales, Australia. 30 pp.

ILAC (The International Laboratory Accreditation Cooperation). 2000b. *ILAC-G13: Guidelines for the Requirements for the Competence of Providers of Proficiency Testing Schemes*. ILAC Secretariat, Rhodes, New South Wales, Australia. 13 pp.

ISO (International Organization for Standardization). 2004a. *ISO/IEC Guide 2: Standardization and Related Activities—General Vocabulary*. International Organization for Standardization (ISO), Geneva, Switzerland. 60 pp. (ISO/IEC Guide 2 was supplemented by ISO/IEC International Standard 17000 in 2004).

ISO (International Organization for Standardization). 1997a. *ISO/IEC Guide 43-1: Proficiency Testing by Interlaboratory Comparisons—Part 1: Development and Operation of Proficiency Testing Schemes*. International Organization for Standardization (ISO), Geneva, Switzerland. 16 pp.

ISO (International Organization for Standardization). 1997b. *ISO/IEC Guide 43-2. Proficiency Testing by Interlaboratory Comparisons—Part 2: Selection and Use of Proficiency Testing Schemes by Laboratory Accreditation Bodies*. International Organization for Standardization (ISO), Geneva, Switzerland. 3 pp.

ISO (International Organization for Standardization). 2005. *ISO/IEC International Standard 17025: General Requirements for the Competence of Testing and Calibration Laboratories*. International Organization for Standardization (ISO), Geneva, Switzerland. 28 pp.

ISO (International Organization for Standardization). 2000a. *ISO Guide 34: General Requirements for the Competence of Reference Material Producers*. International Organization for Standardization (ISO), Geneva, Switzerland. 30 pp.

ISO (International Organization for Standardization). 2000b. *ISO International Standard 9000. Quality Management Systems—Fundamentals and Vocabulary*. International Organization for Standardization (ISO), Geneva, Switzerland. 29 pp.

ISO (International Organization for Standardization). 2000c. *ISO International Standard 9001: Quality Management Systems—Requirements*. International Organization for Standardization (ISO), Geneva, Switzerland. 23 pp.

ISO (International Organization for Standardization). 2000d. *ISO 9004: Quality Management Systems—Guidelines for Performance Improvement*. International Organization for Standardization (ISO), Geneva, Switzerland. 56 pp.

ISO (International Organization for Standardization). 2004b. *ISO/IEC 17011: General Requirements for Bodies Providing Assessment and Accreditation*. International Organization for Standardization (ISO), Geneva, Switzerland. 21 pp.

OIE (Office International des Epizooties or World Organisation for Animal Health). 2002. *OIE Quality Standard and Guidelines for Veterinary Laboratories: infectious diseases*. Office International des Epizooties, Paris, France. 64 pp.

OIE (Office International des Epizooties or World Organisation for Animal Health). 2003. *Manual of Diagnostic Tests for Aquatic Animals*, Chapters 1.1.1–1.1.3. pp. 3–26. Office International des Epizooties, Paris, France.

Wiegers, A.L. 2002. The age of competence: An update on the international laboratory accreditation scene for veterinary testing laboratories. *Journal of Veterinary Diagnostic Investigation* 14:89–96.

Wiegers, A.L. 2003. Valid methods: The quality assurance of test method development, validation, approval, and transfer for veterinary testing laboratories. *Journal of Veterinary Diagnostic Investigation* 15:303–310.

Wiegers, A.L. 2004. The quality assurance of proficiency testing programs for animal disease diagnostic laboratories. *Journal of Veterinary Diagnostic Investigation* 16:255–263.

Wiegers, A.L., J.R. Heidel, and A.D. Scarfe. 2003. Demonstrating data and test result validity for aquatic animal health laboratories. *Journal of Aquatic Animal Health* 15(4):287–294.

Wiegers, A.L., A.D. Scarfe, and J.R. Heidel. 2004. U.S. needs national diagnostic lab system to support biosecurity in aquaculture. Global Aquaculture Advocate, August 2004:32–33.

Chapter 8
Disinfectants, Disinfection, and Biosecurity in Aquaculture

G. Russell Danner and Peter Merrill

Abstract

Disinfection and biosecurity are terms frequently used in the health maintenance of aquatic species. These concepts have been integrated into the husbandry of many aquatic organisms at many levels, especially in finfish aquaculture, where these terms have even become part of the vernacular. Nonetheless, a recent U.S. Department of Agriculture aquatic epizootiological survey revealed that a high proportion of individuals involved in aquaculture were skeptical about the benefits of biosecurity (Gustafson et al. 2003). Disinfection and biosecurity may of course be disregarded, often without immediately apparent consequences, but that is a short-sighted philosophy; and protocols making use of the concept of biosecurity in specific ways are very effective at preventing problems, and are cost-effective when compared to necessarily dealing with problems after the fact. This chapter describes the types of disinfectants available, and some of their uses in aquaculture operations across the United States as well as worldwide; and stresses how disinfection, applied both to known and unrecognized pathogens, should be an integral component of any effective biosecurity program.

Introduction

The concepts of disinfection and what has come to be known as biosecurity are not new. Since the beginning of written history, humankind has recorded guidelines for dealing with disinfection and biosecurity, based upon contemporary understanding of the concepts. Throughout history, the concepts of "clean" and "unclean" have become increasingly refined. Today, a disinfectant, also synonymously and generically referred to in this chapter as a germicide, is defined as "an agent that destroys infection-producing organisms" (Blood and Studdert 1988). In contrast, an antiseptic is defined as a substance that discourages the growth of microorganisms, usually on biological tissues. Several factors should be included in an evaluation of a disinfectant. A prerequisite for a disinfectant is its spectrum of effectiveness against pathogens. It is imperative that disinfectants be selected after establishing their effectiveness against specific pathogens rather than adopting a broad, non-specific,

---

G. Russell Danner, corresponding author. E-mail: grdanner@adelphia.net

unfocused, and often, meaningless disinfectant selection criterion of "something that kills everything." In Maine (U.S.), for example (where the authors work), disinfectants are selected based on their effectiveness against a list of endemic and state-regulated pathogens (Table 8.1). Table 8.1, based, in general, on important pathogens of salmonids, was used to help assess the relative risk, mode of transmission, and most susceptible life stages of infection by various fish pathogens at marine and inland, public and private fish hatcheries in Maine. Globally, pathogens species differ and vary in importance and prevalence. A similar table of locally important pathogens should be constructed as part of a disinfectant selection process.

Since a single product is unlikely to satisfy all disinfection requirements in a given facility, realistic use of disinfectants will depend on the consideration of multiple factors, including the degree of microbial killing required, the nature and composition of the surface, item, or device to be treated, and the cost, safety, and ease of use of the available agents. Appropriate products with a high degree of potency to deal with specific applications should be selected, where possible, rather than selecting a single disinfectant based on its convenience.

Another important factor in the selection of disinfectants that deserves specific mention is disposal. There is no globally uniform disinfectant disposal policy. It is incumbent upon the user to comply with local regulations regarding disinfectant use and subsequent disposal into the environment. Failure to comply with appropriate use and disposal regulations may result in criminal or civil punishment, personal injury, damage to the local ecosystem, and potentially unintended damage to nearby aquaculture or fisheries.

The discharge of disinfectants into the environment is regulated in the United States by both the Food and Drug Administration (FDA) and the Environmental Protection Agency (EPA). Additionally, individual states have departments that may apply stricter restrictions on disinfectant use and discharge.

Similarly in Europe, Japan, China, South America, and Australia, there are specific regulations regarding the availability, proper use, and disposal of specific disinfectants. At the end of this chapter, Internet links to other regulatory authorities in charge of disinfectants

Table 8.1 Efficacy and characteristics of commonly used disinfectants. (From Murray et al. 1999)

			Active against					
Germicide	Use dilution	Level of disinfection	Bacteria	Lipophilic virus	Fungi	Hydrophilic viruses	*M. tuberculosis*	Bacterial 1 spore
Formaldehyde	2–3.2%	High	+	+	+	+	+	+
Hydrogen peroxide	3–25%	High	+	+	+	+	+	V
Chlorine	100–1,000 ppm Cl	High	+	+	+	+	+	V
Isopropyl alcohol	60–95%	Intermediate	+	+	+	V	+	–
Glucoprotamine	4%	Intermediate	+	+	+	+	+	–
Phenolic compounds	0.4–5% aqueous	Intermediate	+	+	+	V	+	–
Iodophors	30–50 ppm	Intermediate	+	+	+	+	V	–
Quaternary ammonium compounds	Active I 0.4–1.5% aqueous	Low	V	+	V	–	–	–

Note: + = yes; – = no; V = variable results. The efficacies of the disinfectants are based on exposure

around the world have been provided. The authors provide these addresses and links, rather than attempt to describe various foreign regulations.

US regulatory framework for disinfectants and sterilants

Kohn et al. (2003) describe the U.S. regulatory framework for disinfectants and sterilants. All personnel using disinfectants in aquatic settings should be aware of federal laws and regulations that govern the sale, distribution, and in particular, the use of liquid chemical disinfectant and sterilant products. Disinfectant applicants should also understand the relative roles of the EPA, the FDA, the Occupational Safety and Health Administration (OSHA), and the Centers for Disease Control (CDC).

In the United States, liquid chemical germicides (disinfectants) are regulated by the EPA and the FDA (FDA/EPA 1993; FDA 1994, 2000). In health-care settings, the EPA regulates disinfectants that are used on environmental surfaces (housekeeping and clinical contact surfaces), and the FDA regulates liquid chemical sterilants/high-level disinfectants (e.g., glutaraldehyde, hydrogen peroxide, and peracetic acid) used on critical and semi-critical patient-care devices. In the past, the EPA was responsible for monitoring disinfectants sold in the United States under authority of the Federal Insecticide, Fungicide, and Rodenticide Act (FIFRA). A label with an EPA registration number became the standard by which to choose a disinfectant. A new law was passed in 1999 that transferred regulatory authority over the sterilants/high-level disinfectants from the EPA to the FDA. As a result, the sterilants/high-level disinfectants will no longer carry an EPA registration number. While the FDA will clear these products for the market, it is still investigating the implications. It is unclear which agency will have the responsibility related to disposal of used disinfectants. Intermediate-level and low-level disinfectants will continue to be regulated by the EPA under the FIFRA, Title 40 of the Code of Federal Regulations (CFR).

The OSHA develops workplace standards to help ensure safe and healthy working conditions in places of employment, and is authorized under Pub. L. 95-251, and as amended,

Table 8.1 (*Continued*)

Important characteristics									
Shelf life >1 week	Corrosive	Residue	Inact. by organic mat.	Skin irritant	Eye irritant	Resp. irritant	Toxic	Env. concern	Typical applications in hospitals
++	–	+	–	+	+	+	+	+	None
+	V	–	V	+	+	–	+	–	Contact lenses
	+	+	+	+	+	+	+	V	Semi-critical devices
+	V	–	V	V	+	–	+	–	Surface areas
+	–	–	–	+	+	–	–	–	Diagnostic equipment
+	–	+	–	+	+	–	+	+	Surgical equipment
+	V	+	+	V	+	–	+	–	Medical equipment
+	–	+	+	+	+	–	+	–	Food preparation and floors

time of less than 30 min at room temperature.

to enforce these workplace standards. In 1991, OSHA published "Occupational Exposure to Bloodborne Pathogens"; final rule [29 CFR Part 1910.1030]. This standard is designed to help prevent occupational exposures to blood or other potentially infectious substances. Under this standard, OSHA has interpreted that, to decontaminate contaminated work surfaces, either an EPA-registered hospital tuberculocidal disinfectant or an EPA-registered hospital disinfectant labeled as effective against human immunodeficiency virus (HIV) and hepatitis B virus (HBV) is appropriate. Hospital disinfectants with such HIV and HBV claims can be used, provided surfaces are not contaminated with agents or a concentration of agents for which higher level (i.e., intermediate-level) disinfection is recommended. In addition, as with all disinfectants, effectiveness is governed by strict adherence to the label instructions for intended use of the product.

The CDC is not a regulatory agency and does not test, evaluate, or otherwise recommend specific brand-name products of chemical germicides, but it has developed certain recommendations for the application of some types of disinfectants. The CDC recommends disinfecting environmental surfaces, or sterilizing or disinfecting medical equipment, and recommends that applicants use products approved by the EPA and the FDA, unless no such products are available for use against certain microorganisms or sites. If no registered or approved products, however, are available for a specific pathogen or use situation, users are advised to follow the specific guidance regarding unregistered or unapproved (e.g., off-label) uses for various chemical germicides. For example, no antimicrobial products are registered for use specifically against certain emerging human pathogens (e.g., Norwalk virus), potential terrorism agents (e.g., *Variola major* or *Yersinia pestis*), or Creutzfeldt–Jakob disease agents.

One point of clarification is needed regarding a difference in how the FDA and the EPA classify disinfectants. The FDA adopted the same basic terminology and classification scheme as the CDC to categorize medical devices (i.e., critical, semi-critical, and non-critical), and to define antimicrobial potency for processing surfaces (i.e., sterilization and high-, intermediate-, and low-level disinfection) (Spaulding 1970). The EPA registers environmental surface disinfectants based on claims of microbiological activity made by the manufacturer when registering its disinfectant. This difference has led to confusion on the part of users, because the EPA does not use the terms "intermediate-" and "low-level" disinfectants, as used in CDC guidelines.

The CDC designates any EPA-registered hospital disinfectant without a tuberculocidal claim as a low-level disinfectant, and any EPA-registered hospital disinfectant with a tuberculocidal claim as an intermediate-level disinfectant. To understand this comparison, one needs to know how the EPA registers disinfectants. First, to be labeled as an EPA-registered hospital disinfectant, the product must pass the Association of Official Analytical Chemists (AOAC) effectiveness tests against three target organisms: *Salmonella choleraesuis*, for effectiveness against Gram-negative bacteria; *Staphylococcus aureus*, for effectiveness against Gram-positive bacteria; and *Pseudomonas aeruginosa*, for effectiveness against a primarily nosocomial pathogen. Substantiated label claims of effectiveness of a disinfectant against specific microorganisms other than the test microorganisms are permitted, but not required, provided the test microorganisms are likely to be present in or on the recommended use areas and surfaces. Therefore, manufacturers might also test specifically against organisms of known concern in health-care practices (e.g., HIV, HBV, hepatitis C virus [HCV], and herpes), although it is considered likely that any product satisfying AOAC tests for hospital disinfectant designation will also be effective against these relatively fragile organisms when the product is used as directed by the manufacturer.

Additionally, few products are specifically labeled for fish pathogens. So applicants must select disinfectants based on specific knowledge regarding the efficacy of the disinfectant on the desired pathogen type. In Maine, it was useful to construct a table of pathogen types (Table 8.2) and compare it to a table of the germicidal characteristics of different disinfectants (Table 8.3), to select appropriate disinfectants for off-label use.

Potency against *Mycobacterium tuberculosis* has been recognized as a substantial benchmark. The tuberculocidal claim, however, is used only as a benchmark to measure germicidal potency. Tuberculosis is not transmitted via environmental surfaces, but rather by the airborne route. Accordingly, use of such products on environmental surfaces plays no role in preventing the spread of tuberculosis. Mycobacteria, however, have the highest intrinsic levels of resistance among the vegetative bacteria, viruses, and fungi. So any germicide with a tuberculocidal claim on the label is considered capable of inactivating a broad spectrum of pathogens, including such less-resistant organisms as bloodborne pathogens (e.g., HBV, HCV, and HIV). It is this broad-spectrum capability, rather than the specific potency of the product against mycobacteria, that is the basis for protocols and regulations dictating the use of tuberculocidal chemicals for surface disinfection. The EPA also lists disinfectant products according to their labeled use, against these organisms of interest as follows:

- List B. Tuberculocidal products effective against *Mycobacterium* species.
- List C. Products effective against human HIV-1 virus.
- List D. Products effective against human HIV-1 virus and HBV.
- List E. Products effective against *Mycobacterium* species, human HIV-1 virus, and HBV.
- List F. Products effective against HCV.

Disinfectant use regulations outside the United States are beyond the scope of this chapter. A list of resources is provided in the Appendix to this chapter, for researching regulations in other locations.

Physical disinfecting agents

Physical disinfectants can be effective tools in fisheries and aquaculture. Physical disinfectants can have advantages that make them more appropriate selections than chemical disinfectants in certain applications. For example, it may be possible to incorporate a physical disinfectant into an aquaculture procedure that provides adequate disinfection and has fewer negative discharge consequences to the environment. This section discusses the properties of several physical disinfectants.

Heat

Heat facilitates disinfection in several ways. Kinetic energy or heat can directly alter biological membranes, and alter ionic and osmotic homeostasis by evaporating water within biological organisms. More generally, chemical reactions are accelerated by increases in temperature (Strus 1997). Increasing the temperature of many disinfection solutions increases the rate of chemical activity, which in turn increases their effectiveness. For example, the initial rate of decomposition of a 1 M hydrogen peroxide (H_2O_2) solution is 3.2 $\times 10^{-5}$ mol L^{-1} sec^{-1} at 40°C, and is slightly more than twice as fast, i.e., 7.2 $\times 10^{-5}$ mol L^{-1} sec^{-1} at 50°C. In many cases, the rate of a reaction in a homogeneous system is

Table 8.2 Classification of certain fish pathogens

Pathogen[a]	Bacteria		Virus		Fungi	Mycobacteria	Bacterial spores	Others	1999 Maine IF&W Fish Health Regulations	Reference
	Gram (+)	Gram (−)	Hydrophilic	Lipophilic						
Infectious pancreatic necrosis virus (IPNV)				X					Yes	Wolf (1988)
Infectious hematopoietic necrosis virus (IHNV)			X						Yes	Wolf (1988)
Viral hemorrhagic septicemia virus (VHSV)			X						Yes	Wolf (1988)
Oncorhynchus masou virus (OMV)				X					Yes	Wolf (1988)
Infectious salmon anemia virus (ISAV)			X						Yes	Roberts (2001)
Bacterial kidney disease (BKD)	X								Yes	Plumb (1999)
Furunclulosis (*Aeromonas salmonicida*) BF		X							Yes	Plumb (1999)
Enteric redmouth (*Yersinia ruckerii*) BR		X							Yes	Plumb (1999)
Proliferative kidney disease (PKX)								X	Yes	Roberts (2001)
Ceratomyxosis (CS)								X	Yes	Roberts (2001)

Whirling disease (*Myxobolus cerebralis*) (WD)				X	Yes	Roberts (2001)
Bacterial gill disease (*Flavobacterium branchiophila*)	X				No	AFS (2003)
Columnaris (*Flexibacter columnaris*)	X				No	AFS (2003)
Aeromonad septicemia (*Aeromonas hydrophila, A. sobria*)	X				No	Plumb (1999)
Coldwater disease (*Flexibacter psychrophilus*)	X				No	Plumb (1999)
Vibriosis (*Vibrio anguillarum, V. salmonicida*)	X				No	Plumb (1999)
Pseudo kidney disease (*Lactobacillus* sp.)	X				No	Plumb (1999)
Streptococcus infection (*Streptococcus innaea*)	X				No	Stoskopf (1993)
Saprolegnia parasitica		X			No	Plumb (1999)

Note: IF&W = (Maine) Department of Inland Fisheries and Wildlife.
[a]Fish pathogens of concern in Maine. Pathogens are identified by type, so that effective disinfection and biosecurity protocols can be developed.

Table 8.3 Transmission and susceptibility characteristics of important fish pathogens

Pathogen name	Pathogen type	Infective dose *S. fontinalis*	Disease susceptibility (High/Med/Low)			
			Eggs	Fry	Fingerlings	Adults
Infectious pancreatic necrosis virus (IPNV)	Virus	10^3	H	H	H	L
Infectious hematopoietic necrosis virus (IHNV)	Virus		H	H	H	L
Viral hemorrhagic septicemia virus (VHSV)	Virus		H	H	H	L
Oncorhynchus masou virus (OMV)	Virus		H	H	H	L
Infectious salmon anemia virus (ISAV)	Virus		–	H	H	H
Bacterial kidney disease (BKD)	Bacteria		L			
Furunculosis (*Aeromonas salmonicida*) BF	Bacteria		L	H	H	L
Enteric redmouth (*Yersinia ruckerii*) BR	Bacteria		–	H	H	L
Proliferative kidney disease (PKX)	Parasite					
Ceratomyxosis (CS)	Parasite		–	–	H	H
Whirling disease (*Myxobolus cerebralis*) WD	Parasite		—	H	M	L
Bacterial gill disease (*Flavobacterium branchiophila*)	Bacteria	10^6	–	H	M	L
Columnaris (*Flexibacter columnaris*)	Bacteria					
Aeromonad septicemia (*A. hydrophila, A. sobria*)	Bacteria					
Coldwater disease (*Flexibacter psychrophilus*)	Bacteria			H		
Vibriosis (*Vibrio anguillarum, V. salmonicida*)	Bacteria					
Pseudo kidney disease (*Lactobacillus* sp.)	Bacteria	10^6	–	–	–	H
Streptococcus infection (*Streptococcus innaea*)	Bacteria					
Saprolegnia parasitica	Fungus	1	H	M	L	L

Table 8.3 (*Continued*)

Asymptomatic carriers	Horizontal transmission: Fish to fish cohorts	Vertical transmission: Parents to offspring	Fomites: Trucks, tanks, tools, equip., etc.	Vectors: Humans, animals, and birds	Vehiles: Humans, animals, and birds	Found in Maine	Closest recent outbreak and date
Yes	Yes	Yes	Low	No	Low	Yes	1999 Goodwins Mills, ME
Yes	Yes	Yes	Yes	No	Yes	No	1990s Western USA
Yes	Yes	No	Yes	No	No	No	
	Yes	Yes				No	
	Yes	?	Yes	Yes	No	No	1999 New Brunswick, Canada
Yes	Yes	Yes		No		Yes	1999 Eastport, ME
Yes	Yes	?	Yes	No	Yes	Yes	1999 Cobb. Str. ME
Yes	Yes			No	Yes	Yes	1998 Grand Lake, ME
				No		Yes	
	No	No	Yes	No		No	
Yes	Yes	No	Yes	No	Yes	No	1999 Rhode Island
Yes	Yes					Yes	2000 New Gloucester, ME
Yes	Yes			No			
						Yes	1999 Waldoboro, ME
Yes	Yes	Yes					
						Yes	1999 Waldoboro, ME
						Yes	1999 Gov. Hill, ME
Yes	Yes		Yes	Yes	Yes	No	
No	Yes	No	Yes	Yes	Yes	Yes	2000 All hatcheries

Note: Fish pathogens of concern in Maine (ME). This Table is a general guideline regarding mode of from many sources, not all of which are in agreement. Fish culturists should remember that individual is a dynamic condition depending on the fish species, the pathogen, the culture environment, and the transmission, populations at risk, and closest known occurrence of the pathogen. Information originated species have varying degrees of susceptibility, pathogen virulence changes over time, and diseases husbandry.

approximately doubled by an increase in temperature of only 10°C (Nebergall et al. 1980). Chemical disinfectants are evaluated at specific temperatures. Use of these disinfectants will be most effective if used within a few degrees of evaluation temperatures.

When heat is used as a physical disinfectant, it can be applied effectively by submerging fomes in heated water, within the confined space of an autoclave, or spraying them with steam. Heat coagulates proteins, thereby destroying their functionality. Heating to 80°C for 10 min kills all vegetative microorganisms. It is critical that surfaces being disinfected with steam reach 100°. Anthrax spores are killed by heating to 100°C for 10 min. *Clostridium botulinum* and *C. subtilis* spores, however, withstand boiling for hours.

Steam cleaning was applied to marine Atlantic salmon *Salmo salar* net pens as part of the infectious salmon anemia (ISA) disease outbreak in Maine in 2001 (Fig. 8.1). Steam was chosen as a disinfectant, not only for its effectiveness against enveloped viruses like the ISA virus, but also because of the environmental concerns about discharging large amounts of chemical disinfectants into the marine environment.

Pasteurization is a specialized application of moist heat generally used for liquids. Pasteurization does not kill all microorganisms in pasteurized liquids. It reduces the bacterial contamination of the liquid without altering the flavor or nutritional quality of the liquid

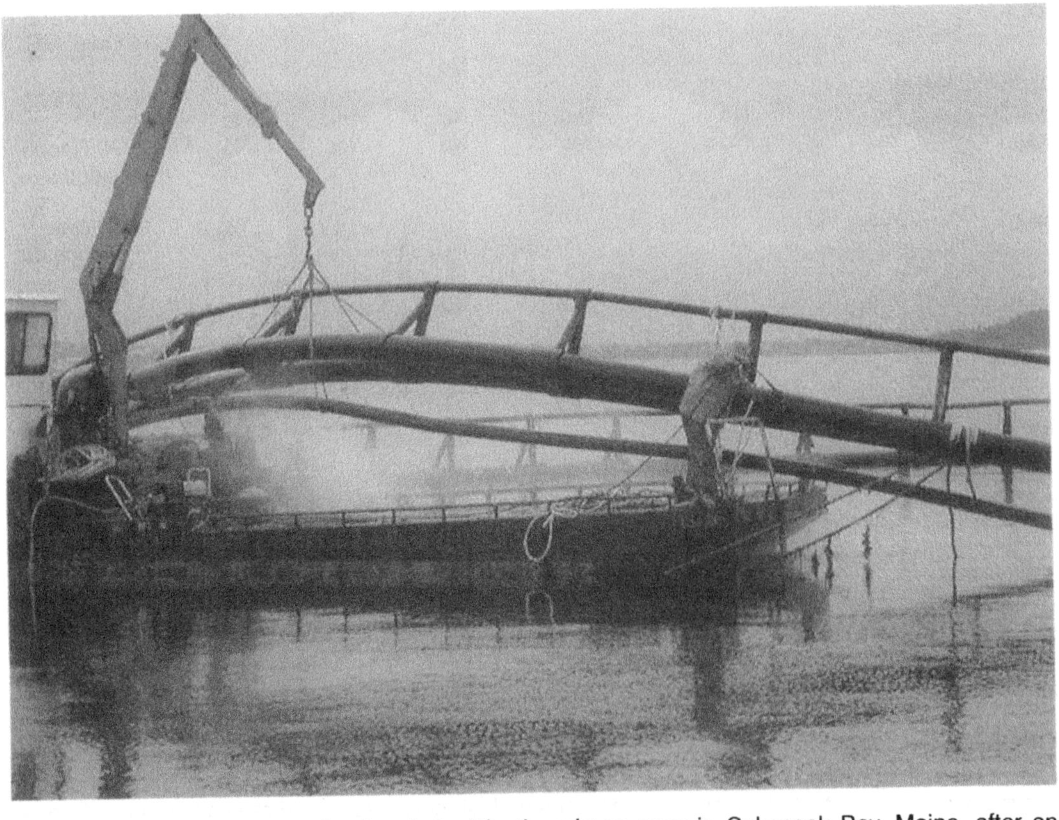

Fig. 8.1 Steam disinfection of polar circle Atlantic salmon cage in Cobscook Bay, Maine, after an infectious salmon anemia outbreak. Photograph by Steve Ellis.

more than necessary. Beverage pasteurization focuses primarily on destroying *Mycobacterium bovis*, *Brucella abortus*, *Salmonella* spp., and *Escherichia coli* rather than sterilizing liquids.

Autoclave is an apparatus for the sterilization of fomes by moist heat under pressure. The pressurized chamber of the autoclave increases the boiling point of water from 100°C at sea level to 121°C at 1 atm above sea level, thereby increasing its effectiveness. The autoclave chamber allows pressurized steam to flow around each article placed inside. The heated moist vapor penetrates cloth or paper used to pack articles being sterilized. Autoclaving remains one of the most effective methods of destroying nearly all microorganisms. The time and temperature necessary for sterilization depend on the pathogen type, fomes, and their packaging. Fish health necropsy tools are autoclaved at the Maine Department of Inland Fisheries and Wildlife (MDIF&W) Fish Health Laboratory, between fish health inspections, to prevent potential cross-contamination.

Dry heat is applied to fomes (flaming or baking), because a physical disinfectant is generally less effective than moist heat. Vegetative microorganisms and spores can be very resistant to dry heat disinfection. Dry heat has some applications including carcass incineration, biomedical waste incineration, searing, flaming bacterial inoculation loops, and wound cauterization.

Compost utilizes the heat generated by decomposing organic matter to destroy microorganisms. Composting can be an effective method of disinfecting feces and other organic wastes (Sidhu et al. 2001; Vinneras et al. 2003). In well-insulated and well-ventilated compost bins, where temperatures can be maintained between 55°C and 60°C for 3–5 consecutive days, composting is an effective means of destroying many harmful microorganisms. Composting is routinely used in Maine to process Atlantic salmon carcasses infected by ISA virus. Composting is used in the United Kingdom to effectively dispose off carcasses from a variety of fish kills.

Sunlight

Sunlight can be an effective disinfectant if given sufficient time and intensity. It is particularly effective in desiccating aquatic macrophages and other organisms. Sunlight has applications in disinfecting drinking water (Conroy et al. 2001; Backer 2002). The three biologically active spectra of sunlight—infrared, visible, and ultraviolet—contribute to its disinfecting properties. Several factors affect the disinfection properties of sunlight, including intensity of sunlight at the time of exposure, which in turn depends on the geographic location (i.e., latitude), seasonal variations and cloud cover, the effective range of wavelengths of light, and the time of day; the type of bacteria being exposed, the nature and composition of the medium, and the presence of nutritive elements capable of supporting the growth and multiplication of the various microorganisms; the characteristics of the container in which the contaminated water is kept during exposure (e.g., color, shape, transparency to sunlight, size, and wall thickness); clarity of the water (i.e., turbidity), and its depth, both being important factors that determine the extent of penetration of sunlight, as well as the possibility of shielding the microorganisms from its lethal effects. Sunlight is used by the MDIF&W fisheries biologists and the Maine Atlantic Salmon Commission biologists to disinfect large gill and trap nets between uses.

Microwave radiation

Microwave radiation is a form of non-ionizing radiation that can be an effective disinfectant in moist applications. Microwave energy accelerates water molecules, and the temperature of the water increases until it turns into steam. Steam is a form of moist heat disinfection. Microwave radiation has current applications in drinking water purification and general disinfection, especially to kill microorganisms on dentures, contact lenses, and baby bottles (Dixon et al. 1999; Xi et al. 2000; Banting and Hill 2001; Hiti et al. 2001; Goodson et al. 2003a, 2003b).

Ultraviolet light

Ultraviolet light (UV), produced by sunlight and mercury vapor lamps, disinfects by damaging the cellular DNA of microorganisms. Ultraviolet light produces primarily a surface disinfection because it does not penetrate many materials deeply (or beyond 2 m in clear water and less turbid water). It is frequently used in aquaculture to disinfect water (Piper et al. 1988; Wedemeyer 2001). It also has applications in air disinfection, and as a supplemental surface disinfectant for surgical surfaces and microorganism growth media preparation areas (Levenson et al. 1986; Murray et al. 1999; Levetin et al. 2001). Using UV light requires human and animal safety protocols, since skin and eyes can be damaged by exposure to UV light. The MDIF&W has large UV disinfection units at the intakes of several state fish hatcheries that utilize lake water. Disinfection by UV light can be expensive. Light bulbs have a limited life and must be replaced regularly. In addition, disposal of used light bulbs can be expensive, since many contain mercury. At the MDIF&W, bulbs are replaced annually, usually in the springtime, when larval fish are being cultured. With this light bulb rotation schedule, new bulbs are installed with maximum efficiency when needed the most, to protect vulnerable young fry from harmful aquatic bacteria and viruses.

Beta and gamma radiation

Two forms of ionizing radiation, beta and gamma rays, work as disinfectants by breaking the DNA strands of microorganisms. Beta radiation is a beam of negatively charged particles. Beta radiation beams of at least 1×10^6 eV are used to sterilize some U.S. mail. Beta radiation is effective against Anthrax spores. Gamma radiation is a beam of very high-energy photons with massive penetrating power. Gamma radiation can be used to disinfect water, concrete, steel, lead, and even soil (Lumley 1976; Kubin et al. 1982; Polishchuk et al. 1989; Sommer et al. 2001; Aksozek et al. 2002). A dose of 2.5×10^6 rads or 25,000 gray (Gy) can be used to sterilize disposable lab equipment and surgical instruments. The shelf life of some foods can be extended with 20,000–50,000 Gy.

Filtration

A series of filters can be used to remove microorganisms of varying sizes from gases and liquids. Water treatment systems filter water, producing a clean water product. Soils and rocks provide a filter for water as it percolates into groundwater reservoirs. Filtering can be an effective means of disinfecting materials that are sensitive to heat and/or chemical disinfectants. Liquid tissue culture media, which contains many nutritional components that would otherwise be negatively affected by heat or chemical disinfection processes, are routinely passed through 0.25 μm filters to remove microorganisms. Fish tissues collected for diagnostic purposes are homogenized and then filtered before they are inoculated onto tissue culture cells during viral disease testing (AFS 2003). High efficiency particulate air (HEPA) filters are used to filter air in surgical suites, laboratories, industrial processes, and biological confinement cabinets.

Impact

Explosives can be effective disinfectants, but their use is impractical in aquaculture and fisheries. There may be a limited application for impact disinfection in removing nuisance species and other aquatic organisms from small ponds or other bodies of water. The shock wave generated by the explosives kills microorganisms as well as some larger aquatic nuisance species. Use of explosives requires special permits in most locales.

Chemical disinfecting agents

A wide variety of chemical compounds are effective disinfectants. The American Chemical Society provides a Chemical Abstract Service (CAS) that includes a chemical registry. The chemical registry is the largest and most current database of chemical substances information in the world, containing more than 23 million organic and inorganic substances and 43 million sequences. The CAS registry mostly covers substances identified in the scientific literature from 1957 to the present, with some classes (fluorine- and silicon-containing compounds) going back to the early 1900s. Each substance in the registry is identified by an unique numeric identifier, called a CAS registry number (CAS NO.). Chemicals referred to in this chapter have been identified by the CAS NO., to aid readers in obtaining additional information regarding the use and safety of each agent.

Soaps/detergents

Soaps and detergents are effective disinfectants. Soap is a particular type of surfactant that is derived from hydrolysis of oils and fats. Soaps are created through the saponification process, whereby the ester linkage in a vegetable oil or fat is hydrolytically cleaved, creating a fatty acid (i.e., soap). Each soap molecule has a long hydrocarbon chain, sometimes called its "tail," with a carboxylate "head." In water, the sodium or potassium ions float free, leaving a negatively charged head. Soap is an excellent cleanser because of its ability to act as an emulsifying agent. An emulsifier is capable of dispersing one liquid into another immiscible liquid. Thus, while oil (which attracts dirt) does not naturally mix with water, soap can suspend oil/dirt in such a way that it can be removed. Both detergents and soaps are considered to be surfactants.

Surfactants that are not soaps are considered to be detergents. A detergent is a compound, or a mixture of compounds, whose molecules have two distinct regions: one that is hydrophilic, and dissolves easily in water (CAS NO. 7732-18-5) and another that is hydrophobic, with little (if any) affinity for water. As a consequence, these compounds can aid in the solubilization of hydrophobic compounds in water, and usually are optimized for this property. Though soap also has these properties, in general, soaps are not considered to be detergents. Detergents are also commonly known as any cleaning mixture containing surfactants. There are several classes of detergents, including:

- *Anionic detergents (or non-ionic detergents).* A class of synthetic detergents in which the molecules do not ionize in aqueous solutions.
- *Cationic detergents (or invert soaps).* A class of synthetic detergents in which the surface-active part of the molecule is the cation.
- *Sodium lauryl sulfate (SLS) (CAS NO. 151-21-30).* A caustic detergent useful for removing grease. Although commonly included in personal care items (e.g., shampoos and toothpastes), it can cause skin irritation and should not be swallowed.

Detergency refers to lifting soil from a surface by displacing it with surface-active materials that have a greater affinity for the surface than they do for the soil. Both soaps and detergents are effective in removing infectious particles from fomes and destroying them. When dealing with contagious diseases, soaps and detergents are generally used for cleaning, and other products are used as a final disinfectant. Proper cleaning will remove up to 99% or more of infectious material and render the surface visibly clean. A visibly clean surface is absolutely necessary before disinfection will be effective. Cleaning is the most important first step in the process of disinfecting fomes.

Phenols

Phenols (C_6H_5OH) are protoplasmic poisons readily absorbed through skin. Since the pioneering use of phenol and water (carbolic acid) as an antiseptic by Lister, a large number of phenol derivatives or phenolics have been developed and marketed. Today, phenolics make up one of the major classes of disinfectants used in hospitals. Phenolic derivatives originate when a functional group (e.g., alkyl, benzyl, phenyl, amyl, or chloro) replaces one of the hydrogen atoms on the aromatic ring. The three phenolics most commonly found as constituents of disinfectants are *o*-phenylphenol (CAS NO. 90-43-7), *o*-benzyl-*p*-chlorophenol (CAS NO. 120-32-1), and *p*-*tert*-amylphenol (CAS NO. 80-46-6). Addition of detergents to the basic formulation results in products with excellent detergent properties that clean, dissolve proteins, and disinfect in one step. Phenolics in higher concentrations act as a gross protoplasmic poison, penetrating and disrupting the bacterial cell wall and precipitating the cell proteins. Lower concentrations of these compounds inactivate cellular enzyme systems and cause leakage of essential metabolites from the cell. Phenol compounds at concentration levels of 2–5% are generally considered bactericidal, tuberculocidal, fungicidal, and virucidal against lipophilic viruses. A phenol-based preparation (14.7% phenol diluted 1:256 in tap water) produced a reduction in rotovirus similar to that achieved with a bleach dilution (800 ppm available chlorine). In a further experiment, both the phenolic and the bleach were able to interrupt the transfer of virus from disks to finger pads (Murray et al. 1999).

Phenolic compounds are tolerant of anionic and organic matter. They are assimilated by porous materials and leave residual films. The residual films may cause irritation to the skin and tissues. Depigmentation of the skin caused by preparations containing *p*-*tert*-butylphenol and *p*-*tert*-amylphenol has been reported (O'Sullivan and Stevenson 1981).

Their use in nurseries should be prohibited, since hyperbilirubinemia has occurred in phenol-exposed infants (Murray et al. 1999).

Phenols are not commonly used in aquaculture. Phenols have been introduced into aquaria through the unwise selection of creosoted driftwood or the use of phenol-based household disinfectants to clean tanks, substrates, or decorations. Phenols are very toxic to tropical fish. They cause severe corrosive damage to gills, skin, and intestinal mucosa. They are also hepatotoxic. Affected fish show restlessness, aimless swimming, and increased respiratory rates. Increased swimming, followed shortly by spastic staggering and death, will be seen with exposures to concentrations as low as 5 ppm. Recovery is possible only if the problem is noticed very shortly after exposure. Treatment is based on removal of further exposure (Joubert and Pretorius 1991; Stoskopf 1993).

In concentrated solutions, phenols may cause severe burns and, if swallowed, can be fatal. They are effective disinfectants against bacteria and some enveloped viruses, but they are ineffective against bacterial spores and non-enveloped viruses. The substituted phenol, 2-phenylphenol (CAS NO. 90-43-7), which has an unwarranted reputation as a broad-spectrum disinfectant, is particularly effective against *Mycobacterium* spp. that are refractive to many other disinfectants. The effectiveness of phenols is also affected by temperature. Phenols are much more effective disinfectants at temperatures greater than 60°C. Phenols have limited effectiveness in the presence of organic matter and should be used only on pre-cleaned, non-porous surfaces.

Carbolic acid is a solution of phenol in water, made famous as the first surgical antiseptic by the Scottish surgeon, Joseph Lister. Its uses in fisheries and aquaculture are limited due to the toxicity of phenols to fishes; except for preservation of tissues for museums or for histological examination (Megvinov 1981).

Cresylic acid (CAS NO. 1319-77-3) refers to the mixture of *o*-cresol, *m*-cresol, and *p*-cresol. At room temperature, *o*-cresol is a crystal or liquid, *m*-cresol is a colorless to yellowish liquid, and *p*-cresol is a crystal. The "mixed" cresols have a phenolic odor. The *o*- and *m*-cresol isomers are soluble in water and in solutions of fixed alkali hydroxides, and are miscible with alcohol, chloroform, and ether. Crystalline *p*-cresol is soluble in organic solvents, and is volatile in steam. All isomers are flammable when exposed to heat or flame, and *m*- and *p*-cresols are moderately explosive when exposed to heat or flame (Lewis 2004). The isomer *m*-cresol is registered as a fungicide for the control of bacteria and fungi on a variety of ornamental plants, on nut trees, on certain stone fruits, grapes, and olives. Cresylic acid was registered for use as a pesticide. Its use, however, is being restricted in the United States.

Acids

The hydrogen ion (H^+) is bacteriostatic in the range of pH 3–6 and bactericidal below pH 3. Acids are effective against bacteria and enveloped viruses. They are not effective against non-enveloped viruses, with the exception of foot and mouth disease virus, which is particularly sensitive to acids. Acids are not effective against the *Mycobacterium* spp., and only certain acids are effective against bacterial spores.

Mineral acids can be used as disinfectants, but they are highly corrosive. Hydrochloric acid (HCl) (CAS NO. 7647-01-0) is a reasonably effective sporicide. A 2.5% HCl solution has been used to disinfect animal hides potentially infected by *Bacillus anthrasis* spores. Sulfuric acid (H_2SO_4) (CAS NO. 7664-93-9), however, is not an effective sporicidal disinfectant. Remember when mixing acidic solutions that the concentrated acid should be diluted into water. Never add water to concentrated acids, because it can result in a dangerous violent explosion.

Carboxylic acids (RCOOH), often referred to as organic or alkanoic acids, are effective disinfectants and much less corrosive than mineral acids. Citric acid ($C_6H_8O_7$) (CAS NO. 77-92-9) is available in the food industry, and has been used alone or as an additive to detergents to destroy foot and mouth disease virus. Acetic acid ($C_2H_4O_2$) (CAS NO. 64-19-7), available as 5% white vinegar, is also an effective disinfectant. The stability and antimicrobial properties of honey are largely due to the presence and antimicrobial activity of component organic acids (e.g., lactic, formic, malic, gluconic, butyric, oxalic, succinic, tartaric, and pyruvic acids) (Cooper and Molan 1999; Osato et al. 1999; Tovey 2000; Molan 2001; Moore et al. 2001; Taormina et al. 2001; Zaghloul et al. 2001).

Alkalis

The hydroxyl ion (OH^-) inhibits or kills most bacteria and viruses at pH >9. Alkalis are effective against all microorganisms, except non-enveloped viruses and bacterial spores.

Sodium hydroxide (NaOH) (CAS NO. 1310-73-2), commonly called caustic soda or lye, is one of the most common alkali disinfectants. Lye solutions are extremely caustic to tissue and skin. Application of lye requires protective clothing, gloves, and eyewear to prevent injury. A 2% lye solution is sufficient for most disinfectant uses. Unless, however, sodium hydroxide is used at a concentration greater than 5%, it is not sporicidal. Never add water to concentrated lye, because it can result in a dangerous violent explosion.

Anhydrous sodium carbonate (Na_2CO_3) (CAS NO. 497-19-8), or soda ash, is a very good cleaning agent. A 4% w/v solution (454 kg per 11.4 L of water) is used for washing vehicles, and is currently used for cleaning the hooves of horses being imported into the USA. With the addition of 0.1% sodium silicate (CAS NO. 1344-09-8) to protect the aluminum of aircraft, 4% sodium carbonate is the only disinfectant currently recognized for use on aircraft hauling live animals (Wheeler 2003). Hydrated sodium carbonate ($Na_2CO_3 \cdot 10H_2O$), commonly called washing soda or sal soda, is sold as a cleaning agent (CAS NO. 497-19-8). When mixing a hydrated sodium carbonate solution for cleaning and disinfection, it requires roughly three times the suggested weight of anhydrous sodium carbonate to get an equivalent hydrated sodium carbonate disinfectant activity level.

Calcium hydroxide (CaOH) (CAS NO. 1305-62-0), commonly called slaked lime, has been used as a disinfectant and is reasonably effective against many non-spore forming microorganisms. When mixed with water, calcium hydroxide forms hydroxyl ions and liberates heat ($CaO + H_2O \rightarrow Ca(OH)_2 + \text{Heat}$). A 20% suspension is used as whitewash.

Biguanides

Biguanides are a class of disinfectants that are mild enough to be used as antiseptics on skin. One of the most common, chlorhexidine (CAS NO. 55-56-1), has been used in agriculture and veterinary medicine for many years (Boddie et al. 1990). Chlorhexidine gluconate (CAS NO. 18472-51-0), a cationic bisbiguanide, has been widely recognized as an effective and safe antiseptic for more than 30 years (King et al. 1977; Zabbia 1977). Its most common formulation is a 4% aqueous solution in a detergent base. The antimicrobial spectrum includes vegetative bacteria, fungi, and viruses. Bactericidal concentrations cause destruction of the bacterial cell membrane, leading to leakage of cellular constituents and coagulation of cell contents.

Chlorhexidine has been demonstrated to be bactericidal against both Gram-positive and Gram-negative bacteria (Best et al. 1990; Boddie et al. 1990; Bettin et al. 1994; Himathongkham et al. 1999; Oie et al. 1999; Penna et al. 2001; Pietsch 2001; Marchetti et al. 2003). In addition to its rapid bactericidal action, chlorhexidine gluconate provides a persistent antimicrobial action that prevents the regrowth of microorganisms. This effect is desirable when a sustained reduction in microbial flora reduces infection risk.

Chlorhexidine has little activity against bacterial and fungal spores, except at high temperatures. Mycobacteria are inhibited but are not killed by aqueous solutions. It is effective against lipophilic viruses. The antimicrobial activity of chlorhexidine is little affected by blood and other organic material when compared to povidone-iodine. Inorganic anions and organic anions, such as soaps, however, are incompatible with chlorhexidine. Its activity is also reduced at an extreme acidic or alkaline pH and in the presence of anionic and non-ionic-based moisturizers and detergents.

Halogens

Members of the halogen group are effective disinfectants when proper cleaning has been done prior to their application. Halogen disinfectants, however, are totally neutralized by the presence of organic matter, which limits their applicability in many aquaculture situations. Halogen disinfectants are generally most effective at environmental pH <7. Halogens are highly toxic to aquatic animals; so care must be exercised around these animals to neutralize halogen disinfectants, before exposure to waters containing aquatic animals. Sodium thiosulfate can be used to neutralize halogen solutions by mixing 5 moles of sodium thiosulfate with 4 moles of halogen.

Among the large number of chlorine compounds commercially available, hypochlorites are the most widely used disinfectants. Hypochlorite has been used for more than a century, and it remains as an important disinfectant. Aqueous solutions of sodium hypochlorite (CAS NO. 7681-52-9) are usually called household bleach. Bleach commonly contains 5.25% sodium hypochlorite or 52,500 ppm available chlorine; a 1:10 dilution of bleach provides about 5,000 ppm available chlorine. Alternative chlorine-releasing compounds frequently used in facilities include chloramine T, sodium dichloroisocyanurate tablets, and demand–release chlorine dioxide. Demand–release chlorine dioxide, a gas, is an extremely reactive compound, and consequently, is prepared at the point of use. It is largely used in the chlorination of potable water, swimming pools, and waste water. Due to its hazardous nature, chlorine gas is rarely used as a disinfectant. Inhalation of chlorine gas may cause irritation of the respiratory tract, resulting in cough, dyspnea, and pulmonary edema or chemical pneumonitis.

In an aqueous solution, all chlorine compounds release hypochlorous acid, which is considered the active compound. The mechanism of microbicidal action of hypochlorous acid has not been fully elucidated. Inhibition of some key enzymatic reactions within the cell and denaturation of proteins play major roles in killing. Lowering of the pH or an increase in the temperature or concentration increases its antimicrobial efficacy. Chlorine compounds have broad antimicrobial spectra that include bacterial spores and *M. tuberculosis* when used at higher concentrations. Therefore, hypochlorite can be used as a high-level disinfectant for semi-critical items. Hypochlorite is fast acting, non-staining, non-flammable, and inexpensive. Its corrosive effects, inactivation by organic matter, and relative instability, however, limit its use. Although exposure to sodium hypochlorite through direct contact may result in tissue injury, the incidence of injury due to hypochlorite use in fish culture is extremely low.

On clean surfaces, available chlorine concentrations of 100 ppm for contact time of 10 min very effectively inactivate vegetative bacteria and viruses. In general, endospore-forming bacteria, mycobacteria, fungi, and protozoa are less susceptible, and a higher concentration of chlorine (1,000 ppm) is typically required to completely destroy these pathogens. ChloramineT and sodium dichloroisocyanurate seem to have less sporicidal action than sodium hypochlorite. Hypochlorites and other chlorine compounds are substantially inactivated in the presence of blood or other organic matter. The CDC recommends use of a 1:100 dilution (500 ppm) to decontaminate environmental spills of blood and certain other body fluids (Murray et al. 1999). Consequently, items used for patient care and environmental surfaces must be cleaned before the disinfectant is used. The presence of a biofilm (e.g., in the pipes of a water distribution system) significantly reduces the efficacies of chlorine compounds as well. The freely available chlorine levels in solutions of opened containers can decay to 40–50% of the original concentration within 1 month.

Chlorine use presents a constant toxicity concern for aquaculture. Levels of 0.1 ppm that are common in city drinking water supplies are fatal to many fish species (Zeitoun 1977; Brooks and Bartos 1984). Fish exposed to chlorine lose color and develop nonspecific signs of respiratory difficulty because of damage to their gill epithelium. The pattern of mortalities differs with the level of exposure. At post mortem examination, nonspecific branchial epithelial hyperplasia is commonly the only finding. Occasionally, fish affected by chlorine exhibit sunken eyes. There is no suitable treatment for chronic damage due to chlorine exposure. The obvious course is to eliminate further exposure. Immediate application of sodium thiosulfate to the tank will reduce chlorine to chloride extremely rapidly, and is the best remedial action when there is an accidental exposure (Capuzzo et al. 1977; Zeitoun 1977; Zeitoun et al. 1977; Brooks and Bartos 1984).

The EPA recommends that effluents discharged into natural waters have no more than 0.03 mg/L (30 ppb) of residual chlorine when released. In the U.K., there is a presumption against the use of all chlorine compounds in aquaculture by the regulatory agencies because of the risk of production of chloramines, which are both toxic and putatively carcinogenic (Herren-Freund and Pereira 1986; Herren-Freund et al. 1987; NTP 1992; Dunnick and Melnick 1993).

Chlorine solutions should never be mixed with cleaning products that contain ammonia, ammonium chloride, or phosphoric acid. Combining these chemicals will result in the release of a chlorine gas, which can cause nausea, eye irritation, tears, headache, and shortness of breath. These symptoms may last for several hours. If fish culture personnel are exposed to an unpleasantly strong odor following the mixing of a chlorine solution with a cleaning product, they should leave the room or area immediately, until the fumes have cleared completely.

Calcium hypochlorite ($Ca(OCl)_2$) (CAS NO. 7778-54-3), commonly referred to as chlorinated lime, can be an effective disinfectant when used at directed concentration

(30% available chlorine diluted 40 g/L of water; 1 pound [lb] per 3 gallons [gal]). Calcium hypochlorite is a dry form of chlorine that is efficient and easy to use. In solution with water, it is used as a general disinfectant to destroy bacteria, algae, slime, fungi, and other microorganisms. Calcium hypochlorite is used primarily to chlorinate swimming pools, and to disinfect drinking water supplies and sewage systems. It is also used as a sanitizer in a number of food processing, commercial, institutional, and domestic applications.

Aqueous iodine and tincture, used in the past, have largely been replaced by the iodophors (Murray et al. 1999). The risk of side-effects from the use of iodophor compounds, such as staining and irritation of tissue, is smaller, and resorption is lower than that from the aqueous iodine. Iodophors are chemical complexes with iodine bound to a carrier such as polyvinylpyrrolidone (povidone, PVP) or ethoxylated non-ionic detergents (poloxamers). These complexes gradually release small amounts of free microbicidal iodine.

The most commonly used iodophor is povidone-iodine (CAS NO. 25655-41-8). Its preparations generally contain 1–10% povidone-iodine, which is equivalent to 0.1–1.0% available iodine. The active species appears to be molecular iodine (I_2). A paradoxical effect of dilution on the activity of povidone-iodine has been observed (Gocke et al. 1985). As the degree of dilution increases, bactericidal activity increases up to a maximum, and then falls. Commercial povidone-iodine solution at dilutions of 1:2–1:100 killed bacteria more quickly than stock solutions (Berkelman et al. 1982; Gocke et al. 1985). Thus, iodophors must be used at the dilution stated by the manufacturer.

The exact mechanism by which iodine destroys microorganisms is not known. It has been postulated that iodine reacts with amino acids and fatty acids of microorganisms, resulting in the destruction of cell structures and enzymes (Rackur 1985). Depending on the concentration of free iodine and other factors, iodophors exhibit a broad range of microbicidal activity. Commercial preparations have been shown to be bactericidal, mycobactericidal, fungicidal, and virucidal, but not sporicidal at the dilution recommended for use. Prolonged contact times are required to inactivate certain fungi and bacterial spores (Ganaway 1980; Pollack and Iny 1985; Woloszyn 1987; Williams and Russell 1992).

Compared with iodine, iodophors have less severe toxic effects, do not cause irritability, and are less corrosive on metal surfaces. They have little, if any, residual effect. The antimicrobial efficacy of iodophors is greatly reduced in the presence of organic material such as blood or fish mucus. Iodine is less effective against non-enveloped viruses than chlorine (Payan et al. 2001).

At state fish hatcheries in Maine, iodine is used to disinfect a variety of trout (*Oncorhychus mykiss* [Walbaum], *Salmo trutta* [Linnaeus]), charr (*Salvelinus namaycush* [Walbaum], *S. fontinalis* [Mitchell]), and salmon (*Salmo salar sebago* [Linnaeus]) species eggs and it is used in hatchery footbaths (Danner 2000). Surface disinfection of salmonid eggs prevents the transmission of certain fish pathogens from parent to offspring, and prevents the transport of certain fish pathogens on the eggs' surface amongst hatcheries. In the United States, intra-state and inter-state movement of surface disinfected salmonid eggs has been effective in decreasing the transmission of *Aeromonas salmonicida* and *Yersinia ruckeri.* The efficacy and toxicity of iodine to developing salmonid eggs varies with exposure time and concentration (Amend and Pietsch 1972; Chapman and Rogers 1992; Cipriano et al. 2001; Jodun and Millard 2001). The United States Fish and Wildlife Service hatchery manual recommends 100 mg/L disinfection, but it has been the authors' experience that salmonid eggs from fish living in soft water do not tolerate iodophor disinfection as well as eggs from fish living in higher alkalinity waters (Piper et al. 1988; Erdahl 1994; Mann 2000; Wedemeyer 2001). In such softer waters, therefore, it is recommended to reduce the iodophor concentration to 50 mg/L, accepting the fact that it may not be as effective, but it is much less toxic. Surface disinfection of salmonid eggs does not prevent the spread of pathogens like infectious pancreatic necrosis virus located on the inside of the egg (Dorson et al. 1997).

Oxidizing agents

Oxidizing agents increase the positive charges on an atom or cause the loss of an electron.

Hydrogen peroxide (H_2O_2) (CAS NO. 7722-84-1) is a strong oxidizer that is used for high-level disinfection and sterilization. It produces hydroxyl free radicals (:OH) that can attack membrane lipids, DNA, and other essential cell components. Although the catalase produced by anaerobic and some aerobic bacteria may protect cells from hydrogen peroxide, this defense is overwhelmed by the concentrations used for disinfection. Generally, a 2% hydrogen peroxide solution is rapidly bactericidal. It is less rapid in its action against organisms with high cellular catalase activity (e.g., *S. aureus*) and especially bacterial spores. Killing of spores is greatly enhanced by increased concentration or temperature. Hydrogen peroxide also acts synergistically with some chemical agents such as peracetic acid.

Hydrogen peroxide has low levels of toxicity to humans and the environment. It is neither carcinogenic nor mutagenic. Concentrated solutions may irritate the eyes, skin, and mucous membranes. Hydrogen peroxide can be easily destroyed by heat or by the enzymes, catalase and peroxidase, to give the innocuous products, oxygen and water. Therefore, it is environmentally safe (Murray et al. 1999). When used as an oxidizing agent, it has an advantage over other oxidizing agents, because the only by-product of the oxidizing reaction is water.

Pure hydrogen peroxide is a colorless, syrupy liquid with a sharp odor and an astringent taste. It has a density of 1.438 g/cm^3 at 20°C, boils at 62.8°C at 21 torr, and freezes at 1.70°C. A 3% solution of hydrogen peroxide is used in homes as a mild antiseptic, a deodorizer, and a germicide; a somewhat more concentrated solution is used as a bleach for hair. A 30% solution of hydrogen peroxide is commonly used in the laboratory as an oxidizing agent. In commerce, the principal usage of hydrogen peroxide is as an oxidizing agent, particularly as a bleaching agent. It is often used to bleach substances of animal origin, such as wool and hair. At present, most cotton cloth is bleached with hydrogen peroxide, because of the innocuous character of the decomposition products and the permanency of the whiteness produced by the peroxide bleaching. A 90% hydrogen peroxide solution is used as a rocket fuel (Nebergall et al. 1980).

Peracetic acid

In its pure form, peracetic acid ($CH_3C(O)OOH$) (CAS NO. 79-21-0) is an extremely shock-sensitive explosive. It is supplied as a 40% solution in acetic acid, which has an open cup flash point of 40.5°C, and it will spontaneously explode when heated to 110°C. Very few disinfectant formulations, and none for fish use, are supplied above 5% peracetic, as it is more dangerous to handle; and above 5%, international law requires special and very extreme hazardous chemical transport precautions. Modern stabilized disinfectants using peracetic acid are generally mixtures of peracetic acid, hydrogen peroxide, and acetic acid. The level of active ingredients in mixed peracetic acid disinfectant solutions is generally 0.25% or less. Peracetic acid, alone or with hydrogen peroxide, is one of the high-level disinfectants cleared by the FDA for processing reusable medical and dental devices. Peracetic acid is an effective sporicide (Wheeler 2003).

Virkon S®

Virkon S® (DuPont Animal Health Solutions, formerly Antec International Limited, Sudbury, Suffolk, U.K.; Product #3001143) is a buffered potassium peroxymonosulfate compound modified with the addition of surfactants and organic acids. It is very convenient to handle, because it is supplied as a water-miscible powder. In a 1% solution, it has a pH of 2.6, and thus would be effective as an acid disinfectant if this were its only mode of action. With the additional activity of the oxidizer, it can be expected to be effective as a disinfectant over a broad spectrum of organisms. The Material Safety Data Sheet (MSDS) indicates that in a 1% solution, Virkon S® is non-irritating to skin or eyes. There is no occupational exposure limit (OES) specified on the MSDS. In Europe, OES levels are only given for chemicals classified as significant by the Health and Safety Authorities. Generally, safe formulations do not have OES assigned, unless the manufacturer chooses to add them. DuPont, who manufactures Virkon, says there is no need. Company literature indicates that at dilutions encountered in normal working solutions, the ingredients are decomposed or biodegraded, and are comparatively harmless (Wheeler 2003). Under European Union law on hazardous chemicals, Virkon is described only as irritant, not corrosive. According to the company website (DAHS 2005), the 1% solution has a 10% loss of initial activity after 7 days in 350 ppm hard water, and the powder form has a 2.3% loss of initial activity after 36 months at 20°C (68°F). Packages of dipsticks are available to check the strength of working solutions of this product. The powder is corrosive and will cause skin burns and irreversible eye damage. It is harmful if swallowed, absorbed through the skin, or inhaled. Users are advised to wear impervious gloves, goggles, and respiratory protection when handling the powder. Virkon S® in its powder form should not be subjected to high temperatures; because when the dry form is heated to 70°C, it decomposes, with evolution of sulfur dioxide gas, which is very toxic and irritating to skin and eyes; but most other chemical disinfectants when heated to 70°C, would give off some type of noxious vapors too.

Virkon is one of the few fish disinfectants with full efficacy data from independent laboratories, for virtually all fish pathogens. It is also fast acting and, of particular importance for fish, works well at low temperatures. Glutaraldehyde and QAC products show poor efficacy at, e.g., 4°C, while Virkon is active in seawater below 0°C, and indeed is now incorporated in ice for biosecure transport of carcasses to processing factories. Virkon has many advantages when used properly in aquaculture biosecurity and disinfection protocols.

Aldehydes

Aldehydes are chemical compounds with the general formula (RCHO). The R group may be aliphatic or aromatic. The aldehydes contain a carbonyl group. It is the carbonyl group that determines the chemistry of aldehydes. The aldehydes are very effective against bacteria and enveloped viruses. They are effective against non-enveloped viruses, bacterial spores, and acid-fast bacteria (Wheeler 2003).

Formaldehyde (HCHO) (CAS NO. 50-00-0) is manufactured by mixing methanol (CH_4O) (CAS NO. 67-56-1) and air, and then passing the mixture through a heated tube containing either silver or a mixture of iron powder and molybdenum oxide. Formaldehyde is a colorless gas with a pungent and irritating odor; it is soluble in water in all proportions. Formaldehyde is sold as aqueous solution that contains about 37–37.5% of formaldehyde by weight, and is known as formalin. The solution also contains 7% methyl alcohol, which is added to inhibit the reaction of formaldehyde molecules with each other to form an insoluble polymer, Bakelite.

Formaldehyde causes coagulation of proteins, making it useful as a preservative of anatomical specimens and in embalming fluids. It is also useful as a disinfectant and as a reducing agent in the production of silvered mirrors (Nebergall et al. 1980).

Paracide-F® has been used since 1909 in the United States in the production of sport, commercial, and experimental fishes. It is used as a therapeutic and prophylactic for the control of external parasites on salmon, charr, trout, catfish (*Ictalurus punctatus* Rafinesque), largemouth bass (*Micropterus salmoides* Lacépède), and bluegill (*Lepomis macrochirus* Rafinesque); and for the control of fungi on salmon, trout, and esocid (*Esox lucius* Linnaeus) eggs. Its use in the health-care setting, however, has sharply decreased for several reasons. The irritating vapors and pungent odor produced by formaldehyde are apparent at very low levels (<1 ppm). In addition, an allergy to formaldehyde can develop in some individuals. The strongest banning of formaldehyde for sterilization and disinfection processes came from agencies of the U.S. federal government, such as OSHA, and the Health and Safety Executive of the U.K. These organizations indicated that inhalation of formaldehyde vapors may pose a carcinogenic risk. The OSHA limits an 8-hr time-weighted average exposure to a concentration of 0.75 ppm in the workplace. Other disinfectants, such as chlorines, glutaraldehydes, hydrogen peroxide, and peracetic acid may replace formaldehyde for the reprocessing of certain medical equipment (Murray et al. 1999).

Glutaraldehyde ($CHO\text{-}CH_2\text{-}CH_2\text{-}CH_2\text{-}CHO$), an oil at room temperature, is stable at an acidic pH and is “activated” before use, by increasing the pH to >7 (CAS NO. 111-30-8). At pH >9, glutaraldehyde decomposes. Organic matter has little effect on the disinfectant properties of glutaraldehyde.

Surfactants

Surfactant molecules have a hydrophobic and a hydrophilic region. The hydrophilic or polar region has an affinity for water. The hydrophobic or hydrocarbon region repels water.

Cationic surfactants include quaternary ammonium compounds. Wide varieties of quaternary ammonium compounds (quats) exhibiting antimicrobial activities have been introduced in the past decade. Some of the compounds used in health-care settings are benzalkonium chloride (CAS NO. 8001-54-5), Benzyl-C_{12-18}-alkyl-dimethyl ammonium (CAS NO. 68391-01-5), alkyl-dimethyl-benzyl-ammonium chloride (CAS NO. 68424-85-1), and didecyl-dimethyl-ammonium chloride (CAS NO. 7173-51-5). Quats are cationic surface-active detergents. The biocidal action appears to result from the disruption of the cell membrane, inactivation of enzymes, and denaturation of the cell proteins (Murray et al. 1999; Quintiliani et al. 1999). Quats are non-staining, odorless, non-corrosive, and relatively non-toxic, but they have a limited antimicrobial spectrum. Recent studies have also reported occupational asthma in some individuals exposed to quats (Purohit et al. 2000).

Quat products sold as hospital disinfectants are not sporicidal, and are generally not tuberculocidal or virucidal against hydrophilic viruses. Scientific investigations by the AOAC use-dilution methods have failed to reproduce the bactericidal and tuberculocidal claims made by manufacturers of quats (Murray et al. 1999). Claims made by manufacturers on labels and results from in-house evaluations not verified by an independent laboratory should be considered questionable. The overestimation of the germicidal activity may be related to incomplete inactivation of the compounds tested. In this case, the bacteriostatic activity rather than the bactericidal activity is measured.

Several outbreaks of human infections have been associated with the use of contaminated quat solutions (Hamill et al. 1995; Sampath et al. 1995). In those solutions, Gram-negative bacteria such as *Pseudomonas* spp. and *Serratia marcescens* were found to survive or grow. Footbaths and tool disinfectant tubs at MDIF&W were found with similar live bacteria surviving in the quat disinfectant solutions, until policies requiring frequent exchange of disinfection solutions and proper dilution of disinfectant solutions were implemented. Organic matter, anionic detergents (soaps), and materials such as cotton and gauze pads can reduce the microbicidal activity of quats.

Quaternary ammonium germicidal detergent solutions are excellent cleaning agents. Therefore, they are preferred agents for the cleaning of floors. Based on their limited antimicrobial spectra, their use should be restricted to ordinary environmental sanitation of non-critical surfaces such as floors, furniture, and walls (Murray et al. 1999).

Anionic surfactants are strong detergents but very weak disinfectants. Examples include alkali-metal and metallic soaps, as well as products such as sodium laurel sulfate. Non-ionic surfactants have little disinfectant activity and are probably most important because they reduce the effectiveness of other antimicrobial agents.

Amphoteric surfactants have bactericidal activity over a wide pH range. Amphoteric compounds can behave both as an acid and as a base. For example, with strong acids, aluminum hydroxide (CAS NO. 21645-51-2) acts as a base ($Al(OH)_3$), forming aluminum salts. With strong bases, it behaves as an acid (H_3AlO_3), forming salts containing the ion (AlO_3^{3-}). Amphoteric surfactants combine the detergent qualities of the anionic surfactants with the bactericidal properties of the cationic surfactants. Some amphoteric surfactants have been used as disinfectants in the food industry for many years.

Alcohols

For centuries, the alcohols have been appreciated for their antimicrobial properties. For infection control purposes, ethyl alcohol (ethanol; CAS NO. 64-17-5) and isopropyl alcohol (isopropanol; CAS NO. 67-63-0) are the alcoholic solutions most often used. Their antimicrobial efficacies are enhanced in the presence of water, with optimal concentrations being from 60% to 90%, by volume. The exact mechanism by which alcohols destroy microorganisms is not fully understood. The most plausible explanation of the antimicrobial action is coagulation (denaturation) of proteins, inactivation of enzymatic proteins, leading to the loss of specific cellular functions. Ethyl and isopropyl alcohols at appropriate concentrations have broad-spectrum antimicrobial activity against vegetative bacteria, fungi, and viruses. Generally, however, they do not destroy bacterial spores.

Alcohols possess many qualities that make them suitable both for antisepsis of skin and for disinfection of equipment. They are fast acting with topical application, non-staining, non-allergenic, and readily evaporate. The rapid evaporation is advantageous for most disinfection and antisepsis procedures. The uptake of alcohol by an intact skin and the lungs, when alcohol is used on the skin surface, is so small that health concerns are not justified. Alcohols have better wetting properties than water, due to their low surface tensions. This represents an important feature for skin antisepsis, along with their cleansing and degreasing action. Repeated application of alcoholic antiseptics, however, may cause drying and irritation of the skin. Alcohols are also excellent for intermediate-level and low-level disinfection of small and clean surfaces of objects, equipment, and environment (e.g., rubber stoppers of medication vials, stethoscopes, and medication preparation areas). After prolonged and repeated use, alcohols may damage rubber and certain plastic items as well as the shellac mountings of lensed instruments. Since alcohols are flammable, one should consider their flame-point prior to application near heat or flame.

Heavy metals

Heavy metals are little used as veterinary disinfectants, but there are some examples of their use that might be of interest. Organic mercury kills bacteria and molds, but is ineffective against bacterial spores. Silver nitrate (CAS NO. 7761-88-8) has been used on burns. Zinc salts are mild antiseptics. Copper salts are used as preservatives and as a topic disinfectant, but fishes are very susceptible to even small amounts of copper (Pequignot and Moga 1975; Richards 1977).

Dyes

Dyes such as trypan red, methylene blue (CAS NO. 61-73-4), and malachite green (CAS NOS. 569-64-2, 2437-29-8) were among the earliest types of drugs used to combat microorganisms (Ehrlich and Shinga 1904). Acridine dyes such as proflavine (CAS NO. 952-23-8) and aminacrine (CAS NO. 581-29-3) are used as topical antiseptics, although they are slow acting and ineffective against bacterial spores. Triphenylmethane dyes, such as crystal violet (CAS NO. 548-62-9) and brilliant green (also called malachite green; CAS NO. 633-03-4), are also used as topical antiseptics. Quinones are natural dyes, and some are powerful agricultural fungicides, such as chloranil (CAS NO. 118-75-2) and dichlone (CAS NO. 117-80-6).

Gas disinfectants

Gas disinfectants are chemical substances that are gases at room temperature and atmospheric pressure. Their use in human and veterinary medicine has increased with the demand to have sensitive electronic equipment disinfected between uses.

Ethylene oxide (C_2H_4O) is a flammable, water-soluble gas that penetrates paper and cellophane easily, and is non-corrosive on delicate instruments and electrical equipment. It is commonly used for sterilization of delicate surgical instruments. Some moisture must be present for ethylene oxide to work effectively (CAS NO. 75-21-8).

Propylene oxide (C_3H_6O) (CAS NO. 75-56-9) is less active than ethylene oxide, and penetrates paper and cellophane poorly, so it must be used on items that are not wrapped.

Formaldehyde is a gas disinfectant dissolved in water and methanol. The disinfectant properties of formaldehyde have already been mentioned (see "Aldehydes" section).

Beta-propiolactone (CAS NO. 57-57-8) is a colorless liquid with a pungent, sweet smell with a 15.6°C (60°F) boiling point. Beta-propiolactone is used as a sporicide to sterilize water, milk, nutrient broths, and vaccines. Beta-propiolactone is now used as an ingredient in vaccines, tissue grafts, surgical instruments, and enzymes, as a sterilant of blood plasma, and as a vapor phase disinfectant in enclosed spaces. Its sporicidal action is generally effective against vegetative bacteria, pathogenic fungi, and viruses. It may be carcinogenic to animals.

Methylbromide (CH_3Br) (CAS NO. 74-83-9) is routinely used as a fumigant for soil, grain, and large structures. It is extremely toxic and dangerous to use.

Ozone (O_3) (CAS NO. 10028-15-6) is an unstable, active molecule that releases an oxygen radical. It is used to purify water. It must, however, be completely neutralized before the water reaches fishes, because it is toxic to them (Ritola et al. 2002; Grotmol et al. 2003).

Resistance of microorganisms

Microorganisms have mechanisms to resist annihilation. They may form protective coatings, they may live amongst organic debris, and they may exchange resistance mechanisms. Generally, resistance mechanisms can be grouped into intrinsic and acquired categories. Intrinsic mechanisms refer to the innate ability of a microorganism to resist annihilation. Some organisms produce coatings or live within other cells, for example. Acquired mechanisms refer to the ability of a microorganism to acquire resistance mechanisms from other microorganisms. Resistance of microorganisms could be a separate volume and goes beyond the scope of this chapter. Murray et al. (1999) provide a good review of resistance mechanisms.

Proper cleaning and application of disinfectants

Cleaning is the most important step in the cleaning and disinfection process. If an item or material is not adequately cleaned, the application of disinfectant is a waste of time and money, because soil (e.g., manure, dirt, secretions, and excretions) cannot be disinfected (Wheeler 2003). The cleaning process can be broken down into four steps: dry clean, wet wash, rinse, and dry. After these steps have taken place, the area should be carefully inspected to be sure it is absolutely clean before the disinfectant is applied.

Dry cleaning

Dry cleaning refers to the process of removing all items that cannot be cleaned or that are disposable. The area to be disinfected should be dry cleaned with a shovel and broom. This step will remove all gross contamination with manure, debris, and feed. Begin the process by hauling the manure to a predetermined site for disposal. When the dry cleaning step is finished, there will be no loose dirt, dust, feed, bedding, manure, or any other loose organic material left within the structure. The surfaces will not necessarily be visibly clean when this step is complete, because of organic matter that is tightly adhered to the surface.

Wet washing

All exposed surfaces, cracks, junctions, joints, and mechanical items should be wet washed with a soap solution or detergent. During the wet wash, it will be necessary to scrub, scrape, or wire brush all surfaces vigorously to break down any biofilm that may be present. Scrubbing can be done with rags on smooth surfaces, although commercially available plastic or metal scrub pads are much more efficient. Rough surfaces should be scrubbed with a wire brush to ensure that they are cleaned as completely as possible. Deep cracks, crevices, pits, pores, or other surface irregularities should be given special attention to dislodge accumulated grime. When the wet wash step is completed, the surfaces will be visibly clean. The moisture on surfaces will spread evenly, wetting the surface completely. There will be no beading of moisture, which would indicate the presence of oil or grease.

The wet wash should be done with hot water. If hot water is not available, assign one or more persons to heat water for washing. Soda ash is a very effective detergent material to use in the wet washing step, but the water temperature must be 35°C or higher for the sodium carbonate to dissolve. It may be necessary to build a fire pit with old blocks, bricks, or rocks. Fifty-five gallon (208 L) steel drums cut in half make excellent containers for heating water.

Special care should be taken around electrical equipment. Utilizing a number of independent lighting units and turning off electrical power if there is danger of getting cleaning solutions into fixtures can reduce safety hazards. An electrician should be contracted whenever possible, for removal of thermostats, timing devices, motor controls, and remote sensing equipment, prior to wet washing.

Rinsing

The washed surfaces must be rinsed thoroughly to remove all traces of soap or detergent. Residue of soap or detergent should not be left on the surface because it may react in an unfavorable manner with the disinfectant. When this step is complete, the water film will still wet the surfaces in the absence of soap or detergent, and there will be no beading.

Drying

The rinsed surfaces should be dried to remove all of the moisture. Removing the moisture promptly will protect equipment and surfaces from deterioration. If left in place, excess moisture will dilute the disinfectant that is to be applied to the surfaces. There may be no practical way to compensate for the dilution when mixing the disinfectant. In cool or cold weather, drying can be accomplished by heating the building and circulating air with auxiliary blowers. In hot weather, drying can be accomplished with blowers or fans alone. In confined areas, or on equipment where air circulation from fans is not enough, the use of high-pressure air from a compressor or high volume "leaf blowers" will remove excess moisture, so that drying can take place.

Inspection

All surfaces, junctions, cracks, and mechanical devices in the building should be carefully inspected to ensure that the cleaning process has removed all of the organic matter. Rewash any areas that may require further attention to pass inspection.

Selection of a disinfectant

Using the information provided above, a family of disinfectants should be selected that will be effective against the microorganisms you wish to destroy. In making this choice, the primary concern is that the disinfectant will function effectively in the environment where it will be applied. Most disinfectants will not work effectively in the presence of organic matter, but some are better than the others in this respect. Choosing a disinfectant that works well in the presence of organic matter may have distinct advantages in environments where cleaning has been difficult to achieve (Wheeler 2003).

After choosing a family of disinfectants, determine which companies offer EPA-approved disinfectants that contain the active agent selected. Obtain label information on each possible disinfectant from the Internet to determine dilution requirements, and check to see that the EPA-approved label of the manufacturer indicates effectiveness against the microorganisms of interest, and that its toxicity and environmental effects are taken into account.

Be sure that the products being considered are available in concentrated form so that the material can be reasonably transported. There are excellent products on the market that are supplied only in final application dilution. Choosing such a product would involve the shipment and handling of thousands of liters of solution in the case of a large task force operation. Because of the logistical problems of handling large volumes of liquids, products that are available as concentrates are always preferable. Check with the company or their distributors for availability and shipment information.

Products that are solids in their concentrated form have a number of advantages. Shipment costs are minimized for the amount of disinfectant used when no water is being shipped. Solid products do not freeze in cold weather, which makes the handling and storage much easier. Solid products can be weighed out in pre-measured packets for use in the field.

Dilution

Proper dilution is required for effective disinfection. The dilution of the disinfectant brings up legal, economic, and safety issues (Wheeler 2003).

Legal issues

In the United States, the EPA approves the use of the disinfectant exactly as stated on the label. The dilution listed on the label must be followed exactly, unless there is a Section 18 exemption that allows a different dilution. Failure to follow label directions makes the individual and the supervisor liable. The situation is similar, albeit less draconian in the EU, and this is likely to follow elsewhere too.

Economic issues

Economic issues can best be served by mixing disinfectants exactly as specified on the label. Disinfectants are tested and proven effective at the specified dilution level. The "glug" or "eyeball" method of measuring are unacceptable.

Safety issues

In most cases, higher concentrations of disinfectants are more dangerous to personnel. Proper dilution is a supervisory issue in avoiding occupational injury and health problems. Many of the stock solutions purchased to disinfect fish eggs and hatchery equipment can be very dangerous. Anyone who uses any of the chemicals discussed in this chapter should read the product labels and the MSDS before attempting to use the products. Always wear appropriate safety equipment and follow label directions. Failure to follow label directions is a violation of federal law, and may result in injuries and penalties.

Application

The application of the disinfectant should be done according to label directions. Disinfectant wet time should be observed carefully. A surface to be disinfected should remain "shiny" wet for at least 10 minutes. Merely damp is not adequate. Porous and rough surfaces will require more disinfectant than smooth surfaces. Since a heavy application of disinfectant that runs off and puddles on the floor is not effective or efficient, a second light application of the disinfectant is one way of keeping the surface wet for the required time. Some of the more useful fish disinfectants also have litmus type papers available for use, to show that the correct concentration has been applied to the damp surface.

Downtime

Downtime is a period during which the premises can dry out completely from the disinfection process, and the numbers of any remaining microorganisms can be expected to decline to a point where there is little or no possibility of infection of susceptible animals. The period of downtime (also referred to as fallowing) can begin as soon as the premises can be certified as clean and disinfected. The period of downtime should be at least three times the longest expected incubation time of the disease in question.

After the cleaning process, disinfection provides progress toward complete elimination of an infectious microorganism, and downtime provides further progress after disinfection. It is an absolutely necessary part of the process, because disinfection is not the same as sterilization. Disinfection is intended to reduce the number of microorganisms so that they are no longer infectious. The need to apply a solution of uniform concentration over huge areas, including ceilings, heating ducts, lights, plumbing, structural members, walls, and floors makes it very difficult to ensure that the process is always done to perfection. In salmon farming in the United Kingdom, however, the atmosphere and walls, ceilings, light fixtures, etc., are routinely fogged with Virkon.

Example disinfection protocols

The following are example disinfection procedures from the MDIF&W (Danner 2000):

Equipment disinfection procedure

There are two equipment disinfection chemicals that may be used to disinfect equipments. A chlorine solution of 200 ppm will be effective in 20–60 minutes. This is the cheapest method of disinfection. Chlorine, like iodine solutions, is less effective when organic substances are found in the water. It can also be diluted by contact with air. Chlorine may be obtained as sodium hypochlorite (HTH) in either liquid or powder form. Powder is the more stable form. The amount of chlorine added to water depends on the percentage of available chlorine in the product used. Sodium hypochlorite powder can be purchased with 15%, 50%, or 65% available chlorine. To achieve a 200 ppm solution (1:5,000 dilution), follow the directions below:

- 567 g (20 ounces) of 15% HTH (available chlorine), powder to 40 L (10.5 gal) of water.
- 28.3 g (1 ounce) of 50% HTH (available chlorine), powder to 68.4 L (18 gal) of water.
- 28.3 g (1 ounce) of 65% HTH (available chlorine), powder to 88.4 L (23.25 gal) of water.

Spray disinfection procedure

The second method of equipment disinfection is to use a commercial quaternary ammonium solution such as TBQ® (dimethyl benzyl ammonium chloride, 8% active ingredients). This product is a detergent-based fungicide, germicide, and virucide concentrate when used at a 1:64 dilution for 10 minutes at 20°C (dimethyl benzyl ammonium chloride; CAS NO. 100-44-7). Quats are not the most effective disinfectants, but they are excellent cleansers that are popular with Maine (USA) hatchery personnel, and are used extensively within the state hatchery system (Fig. 8.2). Care is taken to change disinfectant solutions frequently, and mix them to proper concentrations to maximize their effectiveness. The most strategic and efficient way of applying TBQ® is topical application with a garden-type sprayer. The sprayer allows surfaces of the tank to be covered with disinfectant, without requiring copious amounts of water and disinfectant. Because disposal of disinfectants is an important consideration, minimizing the volume of disinfectant used by strategic application has allowed us to avoid filling the tanks with water and then disinfecting the entire volume of water within the tank. Equipment or stocking truck going between stations should be disinfected before arriving at the next station. A good rinse is all that is needed to neutralize TBQ®. All equipment that has been off the hatchery premises, whether to another hatchery or body of water, should also be disinfected before returning to any other hatchery. Any new equipment brought into the hatchery should also be disinfected before use.

Dead fish disposal procedure

Disposal of dead fish, diseased, or even suspiciously moribund fish is a particularly dangerous procedure as they are the repositories of highest concentrations of highly pathogenic

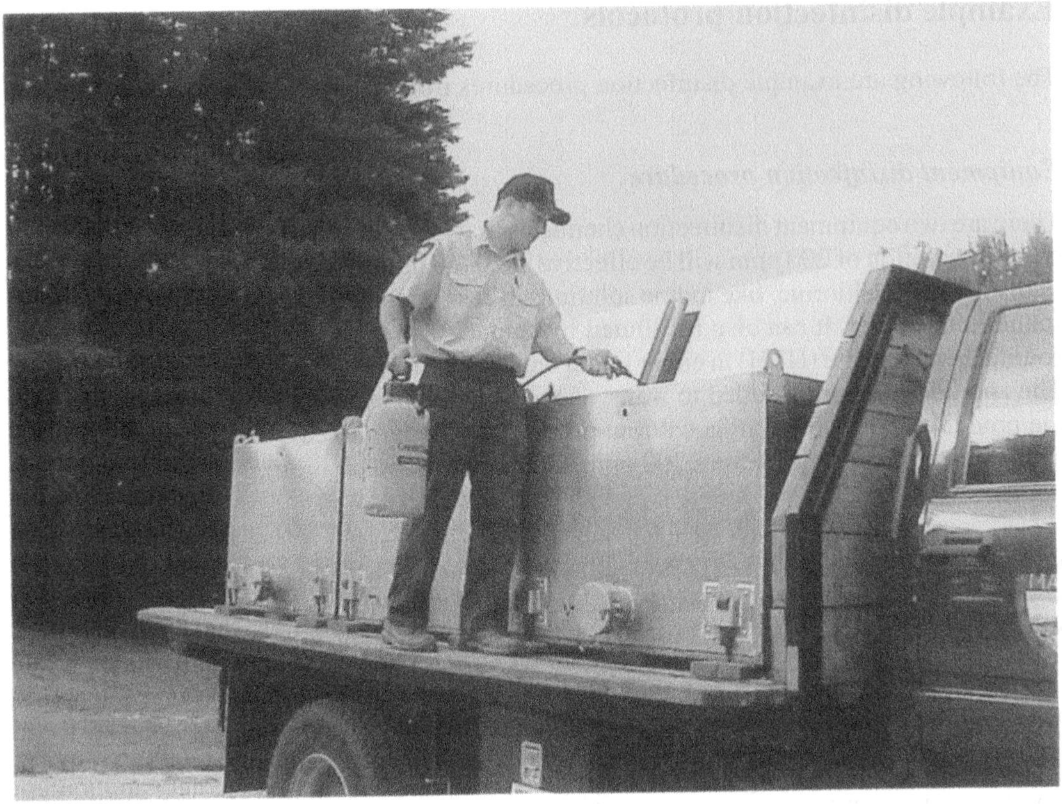

Fig. 8.2 Spray surface disinfection of a Maine Department of Inland Fisheries and Wildlife hatchery truck by a hatchery employee. Photograph by Russell Danner.

agents. They certainly should not be flushed down effluent systems. They should be buried, incinerated, or taken to a proper landfill in sealed bags. Quicklime has historically been used to cover bodies during burial. The use of quicklime can inhibit decomposition of bodies, and decrease the inactivation rate of pathogens in burial pits, so its use in this application has recently been discouraged by the U.S. Department of Agriculture (Jarvis 1997; Bujoczek et al. 2001; Wheeler 2003). Where there are large numbers of dead fish, as for example, following an ISA outbreak in Atlantic salmon, then onshore composting in sealed bins is acceptable, but very high standards of containment and biosecurity around the composting bins are essential until the process is complete.

Footbaths

A footbath should be placed at the entrance to every farm and the doorway entry of each hatchery, in a location easily accessible, and it should be large enough to stand in with both feet and too long to step over without contact. The footbath should contain enough solution to thoroughly wet the sole surfaces of footwear with disinfectant. Footbaths are not boot washing stations. Shoes and boots should be cleaned of excess debris before stepping into or being put into the footbath.

The disinfection solution should be renewed at least weekly (preferably, daily). Everyone entering and leaving the hatchery should step into the footbath, each time through the doorway. Note that a footbath disinfectant that begins the week at 100 ppm will not work properly after the disinfectant concentration decreases with evaporation, dirt, and utilization.

Hatchery visitors

In general, visitors should be discouraged from visiting hatcheries, which are high-tech food producing facilities, at all times. Some public and private hatcheries have biosecurity concerns that make them justifiably closed to visitors. This is the most secure means of dealing with a visitor-related biosecurity threat. Many U.S. hatcheries, however, are required to be open and accessible to the public, a policy that is incompatible with biosecurity. Where visitors are essential, they should be provided with full overall clothing and boots by the farm. Where particularly valuable broodstocks or breeding fish are involved, a full body shower and change of clothing should be provided, as applies in the poultry industry, and in some salmon breeding facilities in Europe and Chile. Biosecurity concerns can be addressed by having consistent written instructions for employees to follow when providing supervised tours of facilities. Common instructions include asking visitors to keep their hands out of the water, and to step into the footbath before entering the hatchery. Visitors may be shown certain areas of the facility, and other areas may be gated or roped to prevent unauthorized access. Effective communication between hatchery employees and visitors about disinfection and biosecurity helps build public confidence in the quality of fisheries and aquaculture products.

Hatchery tools

Biosecurity of each group of fish should be maintained. The practice of moving fish amongst hatcheries exposes staff to potentially catastrophic fish pathogen introduction. Each tank, trough series, or raceway series should have a separate set of hatchery tools. Tools should not be used between different tanks, troughs, or raceways. Tools should be cleaned, disinfected, and stored away properly after each use. Tools for each specific tank, trough, or raceway should be color-coordinated in a simple and easily identifiable manner.

Cleanliness

Keep equipments clean. Dirt, feces, and mud can all harbor pathogens and prevent effective disinfection of equipments.

Stocking trucks, well boats, tenders, and feed barges

Empty vehicles, and clean, disinfect, and rinse tanks with clean water. Fill stocking trucks, transport vehicles, and well boats with clean well water or filtered surface water, tempered to within 5°C of the hatchery water, rather than transporting fish in water from their current container (raceway, netpen, tank, etc.).

Conclusion

This chapter has been written to provide the reader with basic background information regarding the effectiveness of certain disinfectants. Various and numerous organisms can cause disease in fish. Viruses, bacteria, fungi, protozoans, and many invertebrate animals are included in that list. No single disinfectant destroys them all. Effective biosecurity and disinfection should be the key components of any fish health maintenance program. Effective biosecurity and disinfection require identifying the fish pathogens of greatest risk to specific populations, and implementing effective procedures to reduce the likelihood of transmission of these pathogens. Every effort has been made to be accurate, including cross-referencing compounds with CAS numbers, to allow readers to quickly identify compounds and further research them before application.

Acknowledgments

This chapter reviews research results from studies on disinfection and biosecurity conducted in hospitals, dental and veterinary clinics, and by government agencies. Many of the original articles are available through the Internet. The authors would specifically like to thank Kay Wheeler, DVM, formerly of the USDA, for his help and background information regarding many of the disinfectants discussed in this chapter. The *Mortality and Morbidity Weekly Reports* of the CDC on disinfection regulations were also very helpful sources of background information.

References

AFS (American Fisheries Society). 2003. *Suggested Procedures for the Detection and Identification of Certain Finfish and Shellfish Pathogens*, 5th edition. American Fisheries Society, A.F.H. Section, Bluebook, Bethesda, MD. Compact Disc.

Aksozek, A., K. McClellan, K. Howard, J.Y. Niederkorn, and H. Alizadeh. 2002. Resistance of *Acanthamoeba castellanii* cysts to physical, chemical, and radiological conditions. *Journal of Parasitology* . 88:621–623.

Amend, D.F. and J.P. Pietsch. 1972. Virucidal activity of two iodophors to salmonid viruses. *Journal of the Fisheries Research Board of Canada* 29:61–65.

Backer, H. 2002. Water disinfection for international and wilderness travelers. *Clinical Infectious Diseases* 34:355–364.

Banting, D.W. and S.A. Hill. 2001. Microwave disinfection of dentures for the treatment of oral candidiasis. *Special Care in Dentistry* 21:4–8.

Berkelman, R.L., B.W. Holland, and R.L. Anderson. 1982. Increased bactericidal activity of dilute preparations of povidone-iodine solutions. *Journal of Clinical Microbiology* 15:635–639.

Best, M., M.E. Kennedy, and F. Coates. 1990. Efficacy of a variety of disinfectants against *Listeria spp. Applied and Environmental Microbiology* 56:377–380.

Bettin, K., C. Clabots, P. Mathie, K. Willard, and D.N. Gerding. 1994. Effectiveness of liquid soap vs. chlorhexidine gluconate for the removal of *Clostridium difficile* from bare hands and gloved hands. *Infection Control and Hospital Epidemiology* 15:697–702.

Blood, D.C. and V.P. Studdert. 1988. *Bailliáere's Comprehensive Veterinary Dictionary*. Bailliáere Tindall, London, UK. 1123 pp.

Boddie, R.L., J.L. Watts, and S.C. Nickerson. 1990. In vitro and in vivo evaluation of a 0.5% chlorhexidine gluconate teat dip. *Journal of the American Veterinary Medical Association* 196:890–893.

Brooks, A.S. and J.M. Bartos. 1984. Effects of free and combined chlorine and exposure duration on rainbow trout, channel catfish, and emerald shiners. *Transactions of the American Fisheries Society* 116:786–793.

Bujoczek, G., R.S. Reiners, and J.A. Olaszkiewicz. 2001. Abiotic factors affecting inactivation of pathogens in sludge. *Water Science and Technology* 44:79–84.

Capuzzo, J.M., J.A. Davidson, S.A. Lawrence, and M. Libni. 1977. The differential effects of free and combined chlorine on juvenile marine fish. *Estuary and Coastal Marine Science* 5:733–741.

Chapman, P.F. and R.W. Rogers. 1992. Decline in iodine concentration of iodophor during water hardening of salmonid eggs and methods to reduce this effect. *Progressive Fish Culturist* 54:81–87.

Cipriano, R.C., B.M. Novak, D.E. Flint, and D.C. Cutting. 2001. Reappraisal of the federal fish health recommendation for disinfecting eggs of Atlantic Salmon in Iodophor. *Journal of Aquatic Animal Health* 13:320–327.

Conroy, R.M., M.E. Meegan, T. Joyce, K. McGuigan, and J. Barnes. 2001. Solar disinfection of drinking water protects against cholera in children under 6 years of age. *Archives of Diseases in Childhood* 85:293–295.

Cooper, R. and P. Molan. 1999. The use of honey as an antiseptic in managing *Pseudomonas* infection. *Journal of Wound Care* 8:161–164.

DAHS (DuPont Animal Health Solutions). 2005. *Virkon S*®. DuPont Animal Health Solutions, Sudbury, Suffolk, UK. On-line, http://www.antecint.co.uk/main/virkons.htm.

Danner, G.R. 2000. *Hatchery Policy and Procedures Guide*. Maine Department of Inland Fisheries & Wildlife, Augusta, ME. 1100 pp.

Dixon, D.L., L.C. Breeding, and T.A. Faler. 1999. Microwave disinfection of denture base materials colonized with *Candida albicans*. *Journal of Prosthetic Dentistry* 81:207–214.

Dorson, M., P. Rault, P. Haffray, and C. Torhy. 1997. Water-hardening rainbow trout eggs in the presence of an iodophor fails to prevent the experimental egg transmission of infectious pancreatic necrosis virus. *Bulletin of the European Association of Fish Pathologists* 17:13–16.

Dunnick, J.K. and R.L. Melnick. 1993. Assessment of the carcinogenic potential of chlorinated water: Experimental studies of chlorine, chloramine, and trihalomethanes. *Journal of the National Cancer Institute* 85:817–822.

Ehrlich, P. and K. Shinga. 1904. Farbentherapeutische Versuche bei Trypanosomenerkrankung (Article in German, abstract in English). *Berlin Klinische Wochenschrift* 12:329–362.

Erdahl, D.A. 1994. *Inland Salmonid Broodstock Management Handbook*. United States Fish and Wildlife Service, Washington, DC. 141 pp.

FDA (Food and Drug Administration). 1994. *Interim Measures for Registration of Antimicrobial Products/Liquid Chemical Germicides with Medical Device Use Claims Under the Memorandum of Understanding Between EPA and FDA*. U.S. Department of Health and Human Services, Food and Drug Administration, Rockville, MD, USA. 17 pp.

FDA (Food and Drug Administration). 2000. *Guidance for Industry and FDA Reviewers: Content and Format of Premarket Notification 501(k) Submission for Liquid Chemical Sterilants/High Level Disinfectants*. US Department of Health and Human Services, Food and Drug Administration, Rockville, MD. 245 pp.

FDA/EPA (Food and Drug Administration/Environmental Protection Agency). 1993. *Memorandum of Understanding Between the FDA and EPA Notice Regarding Matters of Mutual Responsibility—Regulation of Liquid Chemical Germicides Intended for Use on Medical Devices*. U.S. Department of Health and Human Services, Public Health Service, Food and Drug Administration, U.S. Environmental Protection Agency, Rockville, MD. 5 pp.

Ganaway, J.R. 1980. Effect of heat and selected chemical disinfectants upon infectivity of spores of *Bacillus piliformis* (Tyzzer's disease). *Laboratory Animal Science* 30:192–196.

Gocke, D.J., S. Ponticas, and W. Pollack. 1985. In vitro studies of the killing of clinical isolates by povidone-iodine solutions. *Journal of Hospital Infection* 6(Suppl. A):59–66.

Goodson, L.B., J.W. Bullard, R.T. Glass, and R.S. Conrad. 2003a. A clarification regarding the microwaving of dentures. *General Dentistry* 51:383.

Goodson, L.B., R.T. Glass, J.W. Bullard, and R.S. Conrad. 2003b. A statistical comparison of denture sanitation using a commercially available denture cleaner with and without microwaving. *General Dentistry* 51:148–151.

Grotmol, S., E. Dahl-Paulsen, and G.K. Totland. 2003. Hatchability of eggs from Atlantic cod, turbot and Atlantic halibut after disinfection with ozonated seawater. *Aquaculture* 221:245–254.

Gustafson, L., S. Ellis, and L. Hammell. 2003. Epidemiologic study of infectious salmon anemia in Maine: Combining the subjective and the objective in risk evaluation. Pages 86–98 *in* O. Miller and R.C. Cipriano, editors. *International Response to Infectious Salmon Anemia: Prevention, Control, Eradication*. USDA APHIS Technical Bulletin Volume 1902. USDA APHIS, New Orleans, LA.

Hamill, R.J., E.D. Houston, P.R. Georghiou, C.E. Wright, M.A. Koza, R.M. Cadle, P.A. Goepfert, D.A. Lewis, G.J. Zenon, and J.E. Clarridge. 1995. An outbreak of *Burkholderia* (formerly *Pseudomonas*) *cepacia* respiratory tract colonization and infection associated with nebulized albuterol therapy. *Annals of Internal Medicine* 122:762–766.

Herren-Freund, S.L. and M.A. Pereira. 1986. Carcinogenicity of by-products of disinfection in mouse and rat liver. *Environmental Health Perspective* 69:59–65.

Herren-Freund, S.L., M.A. Pereira, M.D. Khoury, and G. Olson. 1987. The carcinogenicity of trichloroethylene and its metabolites, trichloroacetic acid and dichloroacetic acid, in mouse liver. Toxicology and Applied Pharmacology 90:183–189.

Himathongkham, S., H. Riemann, and R. Ernst. 1999. Efficacy of disinfection of shell eggs externally contaminated with *Salmonella enteritidis*. Implications for egg testing. *International Journal of Food Microbiology* 49:161–167.

Hiti, K., J. Walochnik, C. Faschinger, E.M. Haller-Schober, and H. Aspock. 2001. Microwave treatment of contact lens cases contaminated with acanthamoeba. *Cornea* 20:467–470.

Jarvis, D.R. 1997. Nitrogen levels in long bones from coffin burials interred for periods of 26–90 years. *Forensic Science International* 85:199–208.

Jodun, W.A. and M.J. Millard. 2001. Effect of iodophor concentration and duration of exposure during water hardening on survival of Atlantic salmon eggs. *North American Journal of Aquaculture* 63:229–233.

Joubert, P.H. and S.J. Pretorius. 1991. Laboratory evaluation of B-2 as a molluscicide in the control of the snail intermediate hosts of schistosomiasis in South Africa. *Annals of Tropical Medicine and Parasitology* 85:447–453.

King, J.S., F.K. Neave, and D.R. Westgarth. 1977. Disinfection properties of some bovine teat dips. *Journal of Dairy Research* 44:47–55.

Kohn, W.G., A.S. Collins, J.L. Cleveland, L.A. Harte, K.J. Eklund, and D.M. Malvitz. 2003. *Guidelines for Infection Control in Dental Health-Care Settings 2003 Appendix A. Regulatory Framework for Disinfectants and Sterilants*. Morbidity and Mortality Weekly Report (MMWR), Centers for Disease Control, Atlanta, GA. 62–64 pp.

Kubin, M., J. Sedlackova, and K. Vacek. 1982. Ionizing radiation in the disinfection of water contaminated with potentially pathogenic mycobacteria. *Journal of Hygiene, Epidemiology, Microbiology, and Immunology* 26:31–36.

Levenson, S.M., P.C. Trexler, and D. van der Waaij. 1986. Nosocomial infection: Prevention by special clean-air, ultraviolet light, and barrier (isolator) techniques. *Current Problems in Surgery* 23:453–558.

Levetin, E., R. Shaughnessy, C.A. Rogers, and R. Scheir. 2001. Effectiveness of germicidal UV radiation for reducing fungal contamination within air-handling units. *Applied and Environmental Microbiology* 67:3712–3715.

Lewis, R.J., Sr. 2004. *Sax's Dangerous Properties of Industrial Materials*, 11th edition, Vol. 3. Van Nostrand Reinhold, New York, NY. 4860 pp.

Lumley, J. 1976. Decontamination of anaesthetic equipment and ventilators. *British Journal of Anaesthesia* 48:3–8.

Mann, J. 2000. *Broodstock: Effects of stress and nutrition on egg quality*. EWOS Canada, Surrey, British Columbia, Canada. 3 pp.

Marchetti, M.G., G. Kampf, G. Finzi, and G. Salvatorelli. 2003. Evaluation of the bactericidal effect of five products for surgical hand disinfection according to prEN 12054 and prEN 12791. *Journal of Hospital Infection* 54:63–67.

Megvinov, L.S. 1981. Preparation of anatomic museum specimens while preserving their color and consistency (Article in Russian, abstract in English). *Arkhiv Patologii* . 43:71–72.

Molan, P.C. 2001. The potential of honey to promote oral wellness. *General Dentistry* 49:584–589.

Moore, O.A., L.A. Smith, F. Campbell, K. Seers, H.J. McQuay, and R.A. Moore. 2001. Systematic review of the use of honey as a wound dressing. *BMC Complementary and Alternative Medicine* 1:2.

Murray, P.E., E.J. Barron, M.A. Pfaller, F.C. Tenorver, and R.H. Yolken. 1999. *Manual of Clinical Microbiology*, 7th edition. ASM Press, Washington, DC. 1760 pp.

Nebergall, W.H., H.F. Holtzclaw, and W.R. Robinson. 1980. *College Chemistry*, 6th edition. Health Press, Lexington, MA. 1058 pp.

NTP (National Toxicology Program). 1992. Toxicology and Carcinogenesis Studies of Chlorinated Water (CAS Nos. 7782-50-5 and 7681-52-9) and Chloraminated Water (CAS No. 10599-90-3) (Deionized and Charcoal-Filtered) in F344/N Rats and B6C3F1 Mice (Drinking Water Studies). *National Toxicological Program Technical Report Service* 392:1–466.

Oie, S., A. Kamiya, M. Tomita, A. Katayama, A. Iwasaki, and S. Miyamura. 1999. Efficacy of disinfectants and heat against *Escherichia coli* O157:H7. *Microbios* 98:7–14.

Osato, M.S., S.G. Reddy, and D.Y. Graham. 1999. Osmotic effect of honey on growth and viability of *Helicobacter pylori*. *Digestive Diseases and Sciences* 44:462–464.

O'Sullivan, J.J. and C.J. Stevenson. 1981. Screening for occupational vitiligo in workers exposed to hydroquinone monomethyl ether and to paratertiary-amyl-phenol. *British Journal of Independent Medicine* 38:381–383.

Payan, C., J. Cottin, C. Lemarie, and C. Ramont. 2001. Inactivation of hepatitis B virus in plasma by hospital in-use chemical disinfectants assessed by a modified HepG2 cell culture. *Journal of Hospital Infection* 47:282–287.

Penna, T.C., P.G. Mazzola, and A.M. Silva Martins. 2001. The efficacy of chemical agents in cleaning and disinfection programs. *BMC Infectious Diseases* 1:16.

Pequignot, J. and A. Moga. 1975. Effects of different toxic compounds (Pb, Cu, formol, NH_4) on the carp: Histologic changes in excretory and hematopoietic organs. *European Journal of Toxicology and Environmental Hygiene* 8:361–369.

Pietsch, H. 2001. Hand antiseptics: Rubs versus scrubs, alcoholic solutions versus alcoholic gels. *Journal of Hospital Infection* 48(Suppl. A):S33–S36.

Piper, R.G., I.B. McElwain, L.E. Orme, J.P. McCraren, L.G. Fowler, and J.R. Leonard. 1988. *Fish Hatchery Management.* United States Department of the Interior, Washington, DC. 455 pp.

Plumb, J.A. 1999. *Health Maintenance and Principal Microbial Diseases of Cultured Fishes*, 1st edition. Iowa State University Press, Ames, IA. 328 pp.

Polishchuk, R.F., N.M. Kulinich, and A. Ivanovskii Iu. 1989. Possibility of using gamma irradiation for disinfection of mud and seawater in balneologic practice (Article in Russian, abstract in English). *Gigiena Santariia* 6:65–66.

Pollack, W. and O. Iny. 1985. A physico-chemical study of PVP-I solutions leading to the reformulation of 'Betadine' preparations (5% PVP-I). *Journal of Hospital Infection* 6(Suppl. A):25–32.

Purohit, A., M.C. Kopferschmitt-Kubler, C. Moreau, E. Popin, M. Blaumeiser, and G. Pauli. 2000. Quaternary ammonium compounds and occupational asthma. *International Archives of Occupational and Environmental Health* 73:423–427.

Quintiliani, R., D.F. Sahm, and P. Courvalin. 1999. Mechanisms of resistance to antimicrobial agents. In *Manual of Clinical Microbiology, 7th edition* (Eds, P.R. Murray, E.J. Barron, M.A. Pfaller, F.C. Tenover, and R.H. Yolken). American Society for Microbiology, Washington, DC, USA, pp. 1505–1525.

Rackur, H. 1985. New aspects of mechanism of action of povidone-iodine. *Journal of Hospital Infection* 6(Suppl. A):13–23.

Richards, R. 1977. Diseases of aquarium fish—4: Treatment. *Veterinary Record* 101:166–167.

Ritola, O., L.D. Peters, D.R. Livingstone, and P. Lindstroem-Seppae. 2002. Effects of in vitro exposure to ozone and/or hyperoxia on superoxide dismutase, catalase, glutathione and lipid peroxidation in red blood cells and plasma of rainbow trout, *Oncorhynchus mykiss* (Walbaum). *Aquaculture Research* 33:165–175.

Roberts, R.J. 2001. *Fish Pathology*, 3rd edition. W.B. Saunders, London, UK. 472 pp.

Sampath, L.A., N. Chowdhury, L. Caraos, and S.M. Modak. 1995. Infection resistance of surface modified catheters with either short-lived or prolonged activity. *Journal of Hospital Infection* 30:201–210.

Sidhu, J., R.A. Gibbs, G.E. Ho, and I. Unkovich. 2001. The role of indigenous microorganisms in suppression of Salmonella regrowth in composted biosolids. *Water Research* 35:913–920.

Sommer, R., W. Pribil, S. Appelt, P. Gehringer, H. Eschweiler, H. Leth, A. Cabaj, and T. Haider. 2001. Inactivation of bacteriophages in water by means of non-ionizing (UV-253.7 nm) and ionizing (gamma) radiation: A comparative approach. *Water Research* 35:3109–3116.

Spaulding, E.H. 1970. Role of chemical disinfection in preventing nosocomial infections. Pages 274–254 *in* P. Brachman and T. Eickhoff, editors. *Conference on Nosocomial Infections*. American Hospital Association, Chicago, IL.

Stoskopf, M.K. 1993. *Fish Medicine.* W.B. Saunders, Philadelphia, PA. 882 pp.

Strus, M. 1997. Action of physical agents on microorganisms (Article in Polish, abstract in English). *Roczniki Pantswowego Zakladu Higieny* (Warszawa) 48:263–268.

Taormina, P.J., B.A. Niemira, and L.R. Beuchat. 2001. Inhibitory activity of honey against foodborne pathogens as influenced by the presence of hydrogen peroxide and level of antioxidant power. *International Journal of Food Microbiology* 69:217–225.

Tovey, F. 2000. Honey and sugar as a dressing for wounds and ulcers. *Tropical Doctor* 30:1.

Vinneras, B., A. Bjorklund, and H. Jonsson. 2003. Thermal composting of faecal matter as treatment and possible disinfection method—laboratory-scale and pilot-scale studies. *Bioresource Technology* 88:47–54.

Wedemeyer, G.A. 2001. *Fish Hatchery Management*, 2nd edition. American Fisheries Society, Bethesda, MD. 733 pp.

Wheeler, K. 2003. *Emergency Programs. National Animal Emergency Management System Guidelines. Operational Guidelines: Cleaning and Disinfection.* U.S. Department of Agriculture, Veterinary Service Unit of the Animal and Plant Health Inspection Service, Washington, DC. 51 pp.

Williams, N.D. and A.D. Russell. 1992. The nature and site of biocide-induced sublethal injury in Bacillus subtilis spores. *FEMS Microbiology Letters* 78:277–280.

Wolf, K. 1988. *Fish Viruses and Fish Viral Diseases.* Comstock Publishing Associates, Ithaca, NY. 476 pp.

Woloszyn, S. 1987. Fungicidal effect of iodophor preparations on dermatophyte arthrospores (Article in Polish, Abstract in English). *Polskie Archiwum Weterynaryjne* 27:25–34.

Xi, X., Y. Jin, D. Wu, and B. Ren. 2000. An experiment on disinfection using high power microwave (Article in Chinese, abstract in English). *Sheng Wu Yi Xue Gong Cheng Xue Za Zhi* 17:231–232.

Zabbia, V. 1977. Use of chlorhexidine in surgery (article in Italian, abstract in English). *Minerva Chirurgica* 32:1297–1299.

Zaghloul, A.A., H.H. el-Shattawy, A.A. Kassem, E.A. Ibrahim, I.K. Reddy, and M.A. Khan. 2001. Honey, a prospective antibiotic: Extraction, formulation, and stability. *Pharmazie* 56:643–647.

Zeitoun, I.H. 1977. The effect of chlorine toxicity on certain blood parameters of adult rainbow trout *(Salmo gairdneri). Environmental Biology of Fishes* 1:189–195.

Zeitoun, I.H., L.D. Hughes, and D.E. Ullrey. 1977. Effect of shock exposures of chlorine on the plasma electrolyte concentrations of adult rainbow trout *(Salmo gairdneri). Journal of the Fisheries Research Board of Canada* 34:1034–1039.

Appendix: Relevant Internet addresses

Other sources of disinfection and biosecurity information are available on the Internet.

General information

http://www.biosecuritycenter.org
http://www.oie.int

Fish biosecurity

Australia's AQUAVETPLAN (www.affa.gov.au/content/publications/cfm?objectid=fe5fe7fc-1a49-46-ac661b3270c00b2d&conttype=outputs).
DuPont Animal Health (www.antecint.com/aquaculture).

Safety and personal protective equipment

The National Biosecurity Resource Center, www.biosecuritycenter.org
The National Agriculture Safety Database, http://www.cdc.gov/niosh/nasdhome.html or http://www.cdc.gov/od/ohs/manual/pprotect.htm

Household products

databasehttp://householdproducts.nlm.nih.gov/index.htm

U.S. Federal pesticide laws

http://pmep.cce.cornell.edu/facts-slides-self/core-tutorial/module03/

U.S. Industry

Resources such as the "Biosecurity Guide for Pork Producers" and "Security Guide for Pork Producers", for example, are issued by the National Pork Board in conjunction with the National Biosecurity Resource Center for Animal and Health Emergencies of Purdue

University and the American Association of Swine Veterinarians. Other materials on disinfection can also be found at www.biosecuritycenter.org.

State agricultural extension services

Examples of available information include The Ohio State University Extension Fact Sheets, "Biosecurity for Youth Livestock Exhibitors," "Biosecurity Fundamentals for Extension Personnel," "Disinfection in On-Farm Biosecurity Procedures," "Cleaning and Disinfection of Poultry Facilities," and "On-Farm Biosecurity: Traffic Control and Sanitation." (http://ohioline.osu.edu).

Agricultural Ministries or Departments of other countries

Examples can be found at the web-sites of the U.K. Department for Environment, Food & Rural Affairs (www.defra.gov.uk) (do a search with "disinfectant" as the keyword), and of the Canadian Food Inspection Agency (www.inspection.gc.ca; click on choice of language, "Foot and Mouth Disease," and "Farm Biosecurity—A Common Sense Guide)."

Chapter 9
Aquatic Animal Health Surveillance

F. Chris Baldock, Angus R. Cameron, and Nigel R. Perkins

Abstract

This chapter describes the activities of a surveillance system for aquatic health status on a premises level, and the components of this system. Surveillance activity is important in reducing the risk of the international spread of aquatic animal pathogens as well as control of important endemic diseases. These issues have continued to increase in importance since the formation of the World Trade Organization and the subsequent implementation of various multilateral agreements on trade. Disease surveillance should be an integral and key component of all government aquatic animal health services. It is important for risk analysis, early detection of diseases, planning and monitoring of disease control programs, provision of sound aquatic animal health advice to farmers, certification of exports, international reporting and verification of freedom from diseases, and assurance of pathogen status (e.g., Specific Pathogen-Free stocks). It is particularly important for aquatic animal disease emergency preparedness.

Introduction

During the 1990s, world aquaculture production expanded at approximately 10% per year, between three and four times the rate observed in livestock production over the same period (Lucas 2003). Associated changes in production systems, in particular the trend toward high-density farming systems, have resulted in an environment favorable to the emergence and spread of infectious diseases. Movement of aquatic animals and aquatic animal commodities in vertically integrated farming systems and through expanding global trade agreements have facilitated the rapid spread of diseases within and between different aquatic farming communities. Examples of highly contagious diseases that have appeared during the 1990s include white spot syndrome, responsible for devastating losses in the global shrimp industry after appearing in China in 1993, and viral nervous necrosis, affecting cultured grouper (family Serranidae) in the Asia–Pacific region since 1991 (Reantaso et al. 2000; Owens 2003). Disease is considered as a major constraint to optimal growth of many

Nigel R. Perkins, corresponding author. E-mail: nigel@ausvet.com.au aquaculture species, and is impeding development in many regions of the world (Subasinghe et al. 2001).

Aquatic animal surveillance has an important role to play in reducing the risk of international spread of aquatic animal diseases, as well as the control of important endemic diseases. These issues have become increasingly important since the formation of the World Trade Organization (WTO) and subsequent increased international trade in aquatic animal commodities. As a result, there has been a growing interest in developing better systems for investigating and reporting of aquatic animal diseases (FAO/NACA 2000, 2001; Subasinghe et al. 2001, 2004), and in particular, documenting freedom from diseases that impact trade decisions at regional or national levels. Current international trade agreements, notably the WTO Sanitary and Phytosanitary Agreement (see www.wto.org), and the World Organisation for Animal Health (OIE) *Aquatic Animal Health Code* (OIE 2004), require scientific evidence documenting freedom from disease, before a country can impose sanctions to prevent exposure via imports from countries where the disease of concern exists. Demonstration of freedom from particular diseases can also be used to facilitate market access for exporting countries.

In addition, surveillance is important for risk analysis, early detection of diseases, contingency planning and monitoring of disease control measures, provision of sound aquatic animal health advice to farmers, processors, and other stakeholders involved in the handling of live aquatic animals, certification of exports, international reporting and verification of freedom from diseases, and assurance of pathogen status (e.g., Specific Pathogen-Free stocks). Surveillance is also important for effective aquatic animal emergency disease preparedness.

While the principles of surveillance are common to terrestrial and aquatic animals, there are a number of characteristics associated with aquatic animals that present additional challenges (FAO/NACA 2000, 2001). Aquatic animals present a wider diversity of species, are farmed under varying levels of containment, and often in a far more complex and dynamic environment than terrestrial animals. Aquatic animals are typically farmed in an underwater environment presenting challenges for such activities as observation of behavior, feed consumption, morbidity, and mortality. Diseases often have low or unknown host specificities, and present with non-specific symptoms. Aquatic animals are often farmed under flow-through or open-water conditions making it more difficult to establish health status on a facility or farm basis, in contrast to the situation for terrestrial animals (FAO/NACA 2000). These characteristics, combined with natural migration, movement, and mingling of aquatic animal species indicate that ecological, geographical, hydrographical, and climatological barriers may be more appropriate for defining disease distribution. As a result, the concept of zoning (OIE 2004) has commonly been applied to aquatic animal surveillance and the development of regional or multi-jurisdictional collaboration, to better manage risks associated with movement of aquatic animals (FAO/NACA 2000). Where the distribution of susceptible populations crosses political boundaries, the concept of zonation will be successful only if all affected jurisdictions support the surveillance efforts (Subasinghe et al. 2004).

Disease surveillance and reporting is therefore considered to be a fundamental component of any national or regional strategy on Aquatic Animal Health (Bondad-Reantaso 2004; Subasinghe et al. 2004).

What is disease surveillance?

It is appropriate to define surveillance for the purposes of this chapter, because of the variety of definitions that have been applied by different people over time. The OIE (2003b) *Terrestrial Animal Health Code* defines surveillance as "the continuous investigation of a given population to detect the occurrence of disease for control purposes which may involve testing of a part of the population." This is distinguished from monitoring, which is defined as "on-going programs directed at the detection of changes in the prevalence of disease in a given population and in its environment" (OIE 2003b).

Meah and Lewis (1999) defined surveillance as

> the on-going systematic collection, collation, analysis and interpretation of accurate information about a defined animal population with respect to disease and/or infection, closely integrated with timely dissemination of that information to those responsible for control and prevention measures. (p. 5)

For the purposes of this chapter, the authors prefer the more general definition proposed by Scudamore (2003), encompassing

> the package of activities which provides early warning/prompt detection of animal health and welfare problems, together with tracking and analysis of the way they spread. This process applies not only to infectious diseases, but also to chemical contamination/toxicity, as well as to inherently new diseases. In addition, veterinary surveillance includes animal conditions which may pose a threat to human health—either directly, or via food products—even where such conditions are inapparent in the animal itself." (p. 2)

Purpose and objectives of surveillance

"The primary purpose of aquatic animal disease surveillance is to provide cost-effective information for assessing and managing risks associated with trade in aquatic animals and products (intra- and international), animal production efficiency, and public health. This statement of purpose is consistent with the OIE Code and international perceptions of what disease surveillance is meant to achieve in both terrestrial and aquatic production systems" (Subasinghe et al. 2004, p. 12). The disease focus for a surveillance program in a particular country should include the OIE-listed diseases (OIE 2004), other regional lists of diseases (e.g., the Network of Aquaculture Centres in Asia–Pacific [NACA]/Food and Agriculture Organization of the United Nations [FAO]/OIE Quarterly Aquatic Animal Disease Reporting System, Asia–Pacific), notifiable diseases listed for that country, and any other disease of special concern.

The objectives of surveillance for aquatic animal diseases are

- rapid detection of new and exotic infectious diseases in aquatic animals;
- provision of evidence of freedom from diseases, relevant to domestic and international movement of aquatic animals and products;
- accurate description of the distribution and occurrence of diseases relevant to disease control, and domestic and international movement of aquatic animals and products; and
- assessment of control or eradication success for selected diseases and pathogens.

These objectives are designed to clearly identify what surveillance is meant to achieve, whether the activity be undertaking a survey to describe the distribution and prevalence of an important disease, collecting information to ensure that disease zones are maintained, or assessing success of eradication, fallowing, or other disease control measures. While the term "disease" is most likely to represent an infectious condition, it could also refer to non-infectious causes of illness or loss of production, for example, exposure to a toxin.

Types of surveillance

A variety of names have been used to describe different types of surveillance, reflecting the many objectives for which surveillance is used. Terms such as *passive surveillance*, *active surveillance*, *general surveillance*, *targeted surveillance*, and, more recently, *scanning surveillance* (Scudamore 2003) are used, but the distinction between these terms is not always clear. A brief explanation of terms is given below. More complete discussion of issues surrounding terminology may be found in recent publications (Meah and Lewis 1999; Cameron 2002; Scudamore 2002). A comprehensive surveillance system will comprise a combination of many approaches to the gathering of surveillance data.

Surveillance components have traditionally been classified as either passive or active, in reference to the origin of surveillance data. *Passive surveillance* refers to the secondary use of routinely collected data generated for some other purpose. Types of data include reports derived from diagnostic laboratories, routine field officer activities, research projects, and requests from farmers for assistance. *Passive surveillance* is very useful for early detection of emerging diseases, and often provides a general picture of the disease situation in a population. *Passive surveillance* neither allows reliable quantification of the prevalence, incidence, or geographic distribution of a disease, nor can it be used to reliably demonstrate the absence of a particular disease from a given area. *Active surveillance* involves statistically structured surveys to measure the level of occurrence of a particular disease or pathogen within a defined aquatic animal population. Active disease surveillance includes deliberate and comprehensive "searching" for evidence of disease in a specified population, and, in some instances, provides the data required to prove that the specified population is free of a specific disease. Active disease surveillance programs may be "catch all," i.e., aimed at detecting any significant disease occurrences, or may target specific diseases, or disease control activities. The use of statistical methodology in the design of active surveillance is important to ensure collection of representative and unbiased information. Appropriate analyses can provide valid measures of infection estimates, such as prevalence.

Recent reviews of surveillance in the U.K. have proposed that the terms *passive* and *active* be replaced, because their traditional interpretations were no longer consistent with current activities, leading to potential confusion and misinterpretation (Meah and Lewis 1999; Scudamore 2002). For example, *passive surveillance* has been enhanced in many countries by a range of purposeful activities, and *active surveillance* incorporates activities other than surveys (such as outbreak investigations or testing performed during disease eradication programs). The authors propose that a classification based on the *disease focus* of surveillance activities is more useful, and therefore, the terms *general surveillance* and *targeted surveillance* be used. These terms are defined below and adopted throughout this chapter to avoid potential confusion.

General surveillance refers to continuous observation of the endemic disease profile of a population, so that unexpected or unpredicted changes, or both, can be detected and acted upon as rapidly as possible. General surveillance data may be used to define a threshold level of undiagnosed syndromes that would trigger in-depth investigations to try to characterize them. For example, if gill disease in fish exceeded a given prevalence, this could trigger a diagnostic investigation to determine whether or not this is indicative of a "new" disease. Surveillance of disease syndromes (recognizable collections of clinical signs) could be derived from diagnostic laboratory data or collected from fisheries' officers and harvesters/farmers.

Targeted surveillance collects information on a specific disease or condition, so that its absence can be substantiated or its presence within a defined population can be measured (Scudamore 2002). Targeted surveillance projects may be developed as a result of the findings from general surveillance activities in describing a disease profile. For example, general surveillance in Canadian east coast native oysters (*Crossostrea virginica*), resulted in identification of suspicious histopathology lesions that were subsequently demonstrated to be due to infection with *Haplosporidium nelsoni*, an OIE-listed pathogen of oysters. As a result of this finding from the general surveillance program, a targeted surveillance plan was then implemented, specifically aimed at determining the extent of MSX infections in Atlantic Canada (Stephenson et al. 2003; Subasinghe et al. 2004).

Both general and targeted surveillances are necessary components of a national aquatic animal disease surveillance program. A wholly targeted program is not feasible, because it would be too expensive to carry out surveillance on more than a select few diseases. General surveillance is as useful for the detection of new and exotic diseases, as it is for monitoring outbreaks of endemic diseases. General surveillance increases awareness of disease among farmers and other field personnel, and secondly, establishes working links to expertise providing clinical and preventive health care. Where these elements are weak, or not yet established (e.g., in newly developing aquaculture sectors), there is a stronger case for targeted surveillance. Because resources for targeted surveillance are always limited, risk-based assessments should be used to design effective targeted surveillance programs. If the effort is spread thinly across all aquaculture facilities and sites, then the frequency or intensity, or both, of surveillance will be insufficient for a prolonged period of time. Efforts should focus on facilities, sites, or aquatic populations at greatest risk of exposure to the targeted pathogen/disease.

Basic requirements of a surveillance program

The basis of all good surveillance programs is observant and skilled people with appropriate support resources, who understand what is normal, are alert to changes, and can describe the abnormalities they see. This requires

- appropriately trained and motivated personnel;
- standardized field and laboratory methods supported by quality control systems; and
- access to manuals and training opportunities.

Scudamore (2002, p. 21) has described the process of surveillance as "the collection of relevant information (data) in a structured way (mechanism)." Data are then collated,

Table 9.1 Seven mechanisms of surveillance

1.	Outbreak investigations
2.	Voluntary notification
3.	Compulsory notification
4.	Sentinel surveillance using primary and secondary data sources
5.	Sentinel surveillance using tertiary data sources
6.	Structured surveys
7.	Census

Source: Adapted from Scudamore (2002).

processed, and analyzed to yield information, which is then used to guide decision-making. Data may be described as numerator or denominator data, depending on whether the information relates to cases of disease (numerator), or the total number of animals or farms that could have become cases (population at risk, or denominator).

The seven mechanisms of surveillance are presented in Table 9.1 as described by Scudamore (2002). A brief description of each of the different mechanisms along with advantages and disadvantages is provided in an Appendix at the end of this chapter.

The precise design and structure of a surveillance program will depend on socio-economic and political influences operating at local, regional, national, and international levels.

Components of a surveillance program

Clear purpose and objectives

The four general objectives of surveillance are rapid detection of new or exotic infectious diseases in aquatic animals, provision of evidence of freedom from diseases relevant to domestic and international movement of aquatic animals and products, accurate description of the distribution and occurrence of diseases relevant to disease control and movement of aquatic animals and products, and the assessment of control or eradication success for selected diseases and pathogens.

Objective 1: Rapid detection of new or exotic infectious diseases in aquatic animals

This first objective is considered as an absolute minimum requirement for all countries implementing an aquatic animal surveillance system. It is based on comprehensive general surveillance activities that provide a reference baseline for endemic pathogens within any given area (hydrographically- or oceanographically-based, wherever possible). If this system is working well, new or exotic diseases can be detected effectively using field methods alone (clinical examination and epidemiological description). Levels of diagnostic effort required to identify a new disease have been classified (FAO/NACA 2000; Bondad-Reantaso et al. 2001; Cameron 2002):

- *Level I diagnosis*: Clinical examination and epidemiological description;
- *Level II diagnosis*: Level I in combination with simple laboratory tests such as microscopic examination of blood or tissue samples; and

- *Level III diagnosis*: Levels I and II in combination with sophisticated laboratory tests such as electron microscopy, or with molecular tests such as polymerase chain reaction techniques, or other accepted confirmatory diagnostic techniques.

In addition, diagnosis of a new or exotic pathogen requires use of specific diagnostics, fulfillment of Koch's postulates, integration of epidemiological data, and confirmation from an international reference laboratory. Once a new or exotic pathogen is detected, targeted surveillance will typically be required to define its distribution, the magnitude of the problem and rate of spread, as well as to assess feasible control options, and, where appropriate, demonstrate successful eradication.

Objective 2: Provision of evidence of freedom from diseases relevant to domestic and international movement of aquatic animals and products

Those general surveillance activities that are capable of diagnosing a pathogen or disease of interest may contribute evidence of freedom from diseases of national/international concern. Difficulties have been encountered in incorporating general surveillance information into a reporting system aimed at providing probabilistic or quantitative support for freedom from diseases.

For many diseases, and particularly OIE-listed aquatic animal diseases (OIE 2004), for example, targeted surveillance will be required in addition to general surveillance, to prove freedom from the causative agent. Cameron (2002) describes various methods to ensure comprehensive and scientifically justifiable coverage.

Combining information derived from a variety of sources, including both general and targeted surveillance activities and different levels of diagnostic investigation, is likely to provide the most effective result for surveillance purposes. Simple diagnostics such as clinical or gross examination of affected animals may provide excellent information on disease freedom, for those diseases with characteristic clinical signs and no carrier state. Although this information can rarely provide conclusive evidence of freedom of an exotic disease, more advanced laboratory testing frequently requires validation from simple observations, and either approach is weakened when used as "stand-alone" diagnostic techniques.

It is expected that effective and ongoing demonstration of freedom from diseases will require development of methodologies, allowing combinations of data from a variety of general and targeted surveillance activities in a semi-quantitative or quantitative framework. This is an active area of research and development, and methods are expected to be available within the next several years.

Objective 3: Accurate description of the distribution and occurrence of diseases relevant to disease control, and domestic and international movement of aquatic animals and products

Some indication of the geographic distribution of specific diseases may be obtained from general surveillance activities, provided they are sufficiently comprehensive and include sufficient sample sizes from all geographical areas where susceptible host populations occur. Targeted surveillance, however, involving specific diagnostic techniques (usually

Levels II and III), is usually necessary to provide estimates of level of infection (prevalence or incidence), and more precise geographic distribution information.

Objective 4: Assessment of control or eradication success for selected diseases and pathogens

In some instances, surveillance activities associated with a specific control or eradication program will provide all the necessary information to assess progress for that program. For example, farms enrolled in a disease control program may participate in periodic testing to provide information both for control and surveillance purposes. In an area, however, where some farms are not part of the control program, additional surveillance activities will be needed to determine whether or not the control program is effective with only partial participation.

List of diseases of concern

A minimum list would be those diseases notifiable to the OIE or other available regional lists that are relevant to the aquatic resources or trade interests of a particular country or region. The FAO/NACA list of diseases of aquatic animals was developed specifically for application in Asia (Bondad-Reantaso et al. 2001). Each country may then have additional specific diseases of concern that are added to the OIE disease lists.

Each country should develop a list of diseases that are notifiable within that country, i.e., any occurrence of a notifiable disease must be reported within a specified time frame to the regional/national authority within that country. All exotic diseases for which potential hosts/ecological niches exist in the country should be notifiable. Endemic diseases may also be deemed notifiable under certain circumstances, for instance, diseases under an eradication program, with a defined regional distribution, pathogenic variants of a disease already present in a non-pathogenic form, diseases presenting risks to native flora or fauna, etc.

Information on developing a national list of aquatic animal diseases, and examples of factors influencing the decision to include particular diseases may be found in the FAO Fisheries Technical Papers (FAO/NACA 2000, 2001).

Capability and capacity

A surveillance program must have the capability and capacity to undertake investigations to the required level of diagnostic certainty. This requires planning at local, national, and regional levels with consultation and involvement of all stakeholders. Investment is required in infrastructure, personnel, equipment, and training. Detailed emergency preparedness planning for different possible types of events is an important precursor to mounting a rapid and effective response in the event of a subsequent disease outbreak.

General requirements for aquatic animal surveillance have been described (OIE 2004). Subasinghe et al. (2004) listed four objectives that would need to be met in the development of a national aquatic animal disease surveillance program: improvement in the collection of aquatic animal health information; ensuring sustainable laboratory support; implementation of an information management system; and establishment of national and regional analysis and reporting systems.

It must be recognized that design and implementation of effective and sustainable aquatic animal surveillance systems present a number of challenges, particularly for developing countries. These include varying levels of political, economic, and social development among countries, the transboundary nature of both populations and diseases, variable presenting signs and difficulty in diagnosis for many diseases, lack of effective regulations and legislation encompassing surveillance activities, logistical constraints in applying surveillance activities to flowing and open ocean waters, and lack of health and disease information on many species (Subasinghe et al. 2001). In addition, the developed countries with legislative support, well-developed infrastructure, and resource capacity still report disease incursions (McGladdery et al. 1993).

Data specification

Surveillance involves data collection on a range of different factors, such as specific diseases (number of cases of disease × over a defined time period), patterns of production data, clinical signs or syndromes (e.g., fish deaths, growth rate), and a range of indirect indicators that may be related to disease (climatic factors, insect vector distribution, and water quality). Planning is required to identify precisely what data should be collected under a surveillance program. It is suggested that a "profile" be generated for each disease, syndrome, or indicator that details key information about the disease, data required, and surveillance activities necessary to generate and collect data. Profiles can be stored centrally and made available through a web-based system to field staff, to facilitate review and updating, ensuring that they always contain current information. Profiles should also be developed for non-specific events such as disease outbreaks of unknown causes.

Table 9.2 lists basic information that should be recorded and reported as part of an initial emergency report on a disease outbreak.

Incorporation of GIS capability

Geographic information systems (GIS) offer such a wide and useful range of capabilities that they should be incorporated into all aquaculture surveillance systems. Continued advances in techniques, computing power, software, and increasing availability of data suited to GIS

Table 9.2 Information required as part of an initial investigation of a disease outbreak

- Exact geographical location(s) of outbreak for GIS purposes
- Contact details for affected growers or sites
- Date noticed at initial site and any subsequent sites
- Detailed description of affected animals (history, species, clinical signs, lesions, disease progression, outcome)
- Approximate numbers of affected (sick, dead) and unaffected animals at each location
- Recent movements of animals/personnel/equipment/feed to or from affected sites
- Other epidemiological information: disease in wildlife, environmental factors, etc.
- Preliminary case definition for identifying affected animals and sites
- Preliminary list of possible causes
- Initial disease control actions implemented at the site

requirements have facilitated adoption of GIS in both general aquaculture management (Smith 1999) and veterinary surveillance (Ward and Carpenter 2000; Cameron 2002).

A simplistic description of a GIS is a computer database that handles two broad types of information. The first is geographical information denoting locations for various features such as a digital map (boundaries for farms, regions, or countries; rivers, towns, roads, etc.). The second type of information is called attribute data, describing attributes of geographical features. Attribute data can be linked to one or more features. For example, selecting a particular farm (geographic feature) may allow an investigator to review a variety of attribute data for that farm, such as owner name, contact details, number of animals on the farm, disease testing history, feed available, and so on. Attribute data can be date-linked to allow fish stocks, for example, to be followed over time from their point of origin (breeding farm), through multiple, different intermediate locations or farms, to a processing plant, and even to a market. Attribute data can take any form as long as it represents some form of information that can be linked to a geographic feature.

A major benefit of GIS is the ability to produce relatively simple maps of farms, populations of different aquaculture species (population at risk or denominator data), and farms affected with disease in an outbreak situation. Inclusion of data on populations at risk allows more sophisticated visualization including prevalence or incidence maps, and maps of relative risk of disease. A variety of standardized maps can be automated and made available over the World Wide Web, while more complex maps involving customized procedures or statistical analyses may involve specialized software and expertise. The development of GIS techniques has been complemented by similar developments in statistical methodology for spatial data analysis, allowing incorporation of spatial information into statistical models, to test hypotheses about factors that might be contributing to a disease outbreak (Lawson 2001; Carpenter and Ward 2003; Lawson et al. 2003). In addition, Cameron (2002) describes the use of GIS for spatial sampling, a technique similar to random sampling that involves random selection of one or more locations from an area, as opposed to selecting individuals from a sampling frame. Individuals within the selected location(s) are then sampled, allowing a random sample to be taken without the requirement for a sampling frame, an important capability in a surveillance program.

Developments in computer hardware and software have greatly facilitated widespread adoption of GIS. Desktop computers are now capable of supporting the vast majority of GIS operations. While full-powered, commercial GIS software such as the ESRI® range of products (ArcView, ArcGIS, etc.), remains relatively expensive on a per-user basis, a single copy may be sufficient to support most routine GIS operations for an entire country. Alternatively, a variety of low cost or free software are also available that can achieve much of the functionality of commercial GIS software. Internet access offers a great deal, both as a resource avenue and for collection of raw data and display of GIS outputs.

There are a number of constraints to the implementation of GIS in aquatic animal health. The primary issues are lack of specific skills among users and user groups, and availability of both geographic and attribute data. Training in the use of GIS is easily incorporated into training and support requirements for a surveillance system, and can be adapted to the needs and current skill levels for personnel in any country. In general, it is possible to obtain limited geographic and attribute data without imposing new or expensive demands on surveillance systems or other data providers. It is predicted that availability of GIS data will increase in the future, and adoption of GIS will be greatly facilitated once stakeholders can appreciate some of the potential uses for the methodology. There is a need for short- and long-term training programs aimed at developing GIS expertise among personnel in countries with aquaculture industries.

Data management and reporting

Some form of aquatic animal health information management system is necessary for storing and managing surveillance data and communicating information as required. A national system is required to collect, store, and use the data required to establish and maintain zones. This is principally presence/absence data for mandatory reportable diseases within a country. Data required for risk analysis may be stored at a regional or local aquatic animal support facility (veterinary, governmental, or research), and may be independent of, or linked to, data repositories for surveillance and zoning. Corporate or individual client information may be retained by the direct aquatic animal health service provider (extension officer, local veterinarian, or government aquatic animal health services). Although separate from the national database, this information should be accessible in case of the need to respond to a disease emergency.

The simplest form of aquatic animal health information system relates to the network of individuals involved in the industry (stock managers, feed suppliers, local providers of health care advice), and involves observations and experiences communicated directly by word of mouth. At the other extreme is a national network using computerized data management and analysis systems to link a broad network of expertise including farmers, industry professionals, government agencies, and diagnostic laboratory resources. Involvement of internet-based networks has removed geographic constraints, allowing sharing of information and expertise from all around the world.

National disease reporting system

Special emergency disease reporting mechanisms for *potentially* serious disease outbreaks or incidents are an essential component of surveillance designed to provide an early warning system. These reporting mechanisms allow critical epidemiological information to be transmitted quickly and accurately to the national authorities responsible for aquatic animal disease control. A national disease reporting system should be based on the day-to-day disease investigation activities by field officers and at diagnostic laboratories. Such a reporting system, by necessity, requires feedback loops. An example of information flow in such a system is shown in Figure 9.1. At the first stage of investigation, sufficient data is collected to assist the industry stakeholder with their problem. Only a small proportion of the field information is required by the next administrative level, and likewise "up the line." An audit trail, however, should be maintained of all records generated at each stage of reporting. Thus, although higher-level reports may contain only a very brief summary of each investigation, the full information can be accessed if required.

International disease reporting

There are various international levels of formal reporting, the most important for aquatic animal diseases being through the OIE for all member countries, and the Network of

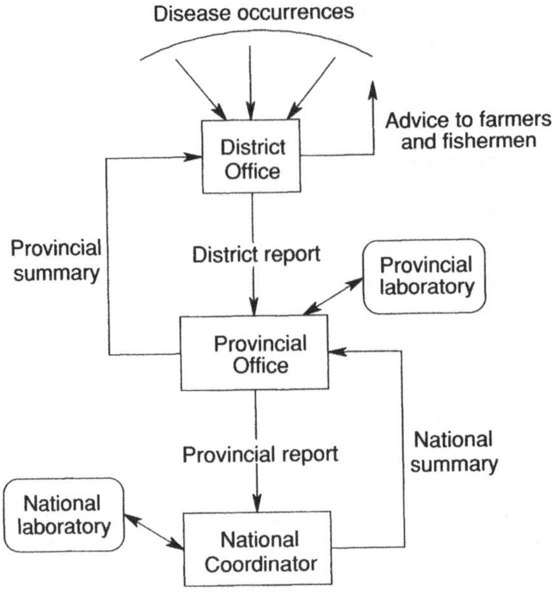

Fig. 9.1 Example of information flow in a national disease reporting system.

Aquaculture Centres in Asia–Pacific NACA/OIE/FAO Quarterly Disease Reporting System for Asia–Pacific countries (FAO/NACA 2001). Of these, OIE has the responsibility for developing international standards for aquatic animal disease control for diseases deemed of international trade importance.

The OIE has obligatory disease reporting requirements for member countries that need to be addressed within any national aquatic animal disease control program. These are outlined in relevant sections of the *Aquatic Code* (OIE 2004) or *Terrestrial Animal Health Code* (OIE 2003b). A staff member in the national office of the competent authority should be delegated the responsibility of preparing draft international disease reports for OIE (and, as appropriate, elsewhere, e.g., NACA, International Council for the Exploration of the Seas [ICES], European Inland Fisheries Advisory Council [EIFAC]), for the approval of the Responsible or Competent Authority. The OIE has recently released new guidelines for aquatic animal surveillance in the *Manual of Diagnostic Tests for Aquatic Animals* (OIE 2003a). These guidelines break free from the previous prescriptive approaches, and enable authorities to use a range of surveillance methods, appropriate to the species, and the environmental and cultural conditions present in a particular region or country. New approaches to the analysis of surveillance data have also opened up opportunities for the use of non-random data to support claims of disease freedom.

A variety of regional organizations have been established to assist international cooperation on aquatic animal health issues, and develop infrastructure to facilitate safe international trade in aquatic animals and their products. These organizations may also have requirements of their member countries, similar to those of OIE, for reporting and sharing of information on diseases, but may include diseases of more regional significance that are not included on the OIE list. The NACA/OIE/FAO Quarterly Aquatic Animal Disease Reporting System (FAO/NACA 2000) is an example of such cooperation in the Asian region.

The NACA/OIE/FAO list includes all diseases listed by OIE as notifiable, as well as the "other significant diseases" listed by OIE and diseases of significance to trade within the Asia–Pacific Region.

In addition, neighboring countries and trading partners may have specific agreements concerning new disease occurrences and the spread of existing epidemic diseases to new areas, particularly near shared borders. Information flows under these agreements may exist at different levels, for example, between the respective National Government Agencies, and also at a local level between contiguous District, State, Provincial, or Regional offices, as well as industry associations along shared borders.

Implementing a basic surveillance program

Most countries could easily conduct a simple form of surveillance based on existing informal communication networks, by adding a formal recording and reporting structure. This would make good use of existing information and provide a historical record of qualitative surveillance information. A central coordinator should be appointed to ensure that surveillance information is disseminated to all interested stakeholders (e.g., through a regular bulletin summarizing the national situation). Potential sources of surveillance information are listed in Table 9.3.

Information sources may be quite varied, and may depend on personal contacts within the local aquatic production community. The types of information may vary from anecdotal information, and unofficial reports (e.g., farmer records, hatchery records, private lab reports, etc.), to official reports (government aquatic animal health reports, certificates, research studies, extension reports), and may be of varying levels of reliability or quality. All

Table 9.3 Potential sources of surveillance information on aquatic animal diseases

Farm/Lease workers
Villagers
Village elders/chiefs
Industry associations
Hatcheries
Buyers/brokers
Markets
Processors/exporters
Post-larvae/fry/seed stock suppliers
Other sales or delivery personnel
Material suppliers
Fisheries officers
Extension officers
Consultants
Research workers
Research institutes
Government/private laboratories
Scientific literature
Non-scientific literature

information has some value, but as the information becomes less reliable, more attention should be paid to verification and confirmation of the information.

Conclusion

Aquaculture production is expanding along with rapid changes in international trading arrangements. Acquiring, analysing, and reporting information on the health of aquatic animals are becoming increasingly important to aid decision-makers in developing a sound policy, not only for disease control, but also for quarantine and health certification, to permit the safe movement of aquatic animal commodities, both within and between countries. Aquatic animal surveillance is a key component of this process.

References

Bondad-Reantaso, M. 2004. Development of national strategy on aquatic animal health management in Asia. Pages 103–108 *in* J.R. Arthur and M.G. Bondad-Reantaso, editors. *Capacity and Awareness Building on Import Risk Analysis for Aquatic Animals*. Proceedings of the Workshops, Bangkok, Thailand, 1–6 April 2002 and Mazatlan, Mexico, 12–17 August 2002. APEC FWG 01/2002. Network of Aquaculture Centres in Asia–Pacific (NACA), Bangkok, Thailand. 203 pp.

Bondad-Reantaso, M., S. McGladdery, I. East, and R. Subasinghe, editors. 2001. *Asia Diagnostic Guide to Aquatic Animal Diseases*. FAO Fisheries Technical Paper, No. 402, Suppl. 2. Food and Agriculture Organization of the United Nations, Rome, Italy. 236 pp.

Cameron, A. 2002. *Survey Toolbox for Aquatic Animal Diseases: A Practical Manual and software package*. Australian Centre for International Agricultural Research, Canberra, Australia. 375 pp.

Carpenter, T. and M. Ward. 2003. Methods for determining spatial clusters in surveillance and survey programs. Pages 101–118 *in* M. Salman, editor. *Animal Disease Surveillance and Survey Systems*. Iowa State Press, Ames, IA.

FAO/NACA (Food and Agriculture Organization of the United Nations/Network of Aquaculture Centres in Asia–Pacific). 2000. *Asia Regional Technical Guidelines on Health Management for the Responsible Movement of Live Aquatic Animals and the Beijing Consensus and Implementation Strategy*. FAO Fisheries Technical Paper No. 402. Food and Agriculture Organization of the United Nations, Rome, Italy. 53 pp.

FAO/NACA (Food and Agriculture Organization of the United Nations/Network of Aquaculture Centres in Asia–Pacific). 2001. *Manual of Procedures for the Implementation of the Asia Regional Technical Guidelines on Health Management for the Responsible Movement of Live Aquatic Animals*. FAO Fisheries Technical Paper No. 402, Suppl. 1. Food and Agriculture Organization of the United Nations, Rome, Italy. 106 pp.

Lawson, A. 2001. *Statistical Methods in Spatial Epidemiology*. John Wiley and Sons, Chichester, England. 277 pp.

Lawson, A., W. Browne, and C. Vidal Roderio. 2003. *Disease Mapping with WinBUGS and MLwiN*. John Wiley and Sons, Chichester, England. 277 pp.

Lucas, J. 2003. Introduction. Pages 1–10 *in* J. Lucas and P. Southgate, editors. *Aquaculture: Farming Aquatic Animals and Plants*. Blackwell Publishing Company, Oxford, UK.

McGladdery, S., B. Bradford, and D. Scarratt. 1993. Investigations into the transmission of parasites of the bay scallop, *Argopecten irradians* (Lamarck, 1819), during quarantine introduction to Canadian waters. *Journal of Shellfish Research* 12:49–58.

Meah, M. and G. Lewis. 1999. *A Review of Veterinary Surveillance in England and Wales with Special Reference to Work Supported by the Ministry of Agriculture, Fisheries and Food.* Ministry of Agriculture, Forestry and Fisheries, London, UK. 128 pp.

OIE (World Organisation for Animal Health). 2003a. *Manual of Diagnostic Tests for Aquatic Animals.* 4th edition. OIE (World organization for animal health), Paris, France. On-line version, http://www.oie.int/eng/normes/fmanual/A_summry.htm.

OIE (World Organisation for Animal Health). 2003b. *Terrestrial Animal Health Code.* 12th edition. OIE (World organization for animal health), Paris, France. On-line version, http://www.oie.int /eng/normes/MCode/A_summry.htm.

OIE (World Organisation for Animal Health). 2004. *International Aquatic Animal Health Code.* 7th edition. OIE (World organization for animal health), Paris, France. On-line version, http://www.oie.int/eng/normes/fcode/A_summry.htm.

Owens, L. 2003. Diseases. Pages 199–214 *in* J. Lucas and P. Southgate, editors. *Aquaculture: Farming Aquatic Animals and Plants.* Blackwell Publishing Company, Oxford, UK.

Reantaso, M., M. Phillips, and R. Subasinghe. 2000. *Developing a Surveillance Program for Aquatic Animal Diseases in the Asia–Pacific: Progress and Constraints.* Abstract 705 *in* 9th Symposium of the International Society for Veterinary Epidemiology and Economics, Breckenridge, CO, 6–11 August 2000. 9th ISVEE Proceedings on CD-ROM.

Scudamore, J. 2002. *Partnership, Priorities and Professionalism—A Proposed Strategy for Enhancing Veterinary Surveillance in the UK.* Department for Environmental Food and Rural Affairs, London, UK. 100 pp.

Scudamore, J. 2003. *Partnership, Priorities and Professionalism—A Strategy for Enhancing Veterinary Surveillance in the UK.* Department for Environmental Food and Rural Affairs, London, UK. 28 pp.

Smith, P. 1999. Application of GIS to the Thai shrimp farm survey. Pages 113–130 *in* P. Smith, editor. *Towards Sustainable Shrimp Culture in Thailand and the Region.* Proceedings of an Australian Centre for International Agricultural Research workshop Songkhla, Thailand, 28 October–1 November 1996. Australian Centre for International Agricultural Research, Canberra, Australia.

Stephenson, M., S. McGladdery, M. Maillet, A. Veniot, and G. Meye. 2003. *First Reported Occurrence of MSX in Canada.* Programme and abstracts of the 95th Annual Meeting of the National Shellfish Association, New Orleans, LA, 13–17 April 2003. 57 pp.

Subasinghe, R., M. Bondad-Reantaso, and S. McGladdery. 2001. Aquaculture development, health and wealth. *In* R. Subasinghe, P. Bueno, M. Phillips, C. Hough, S. McGladdery, and J. Arthur, editors. *Aquaculture in the Third Millennium.* Pages 167–191 *in* Technical Proceedings of the Conference on Aquaculture in the Third Millennium, Bangkok, Thailand, 20–25 February 2000. Network of Aquaculture Centres in Asia–Pacific, Bangkok, Thailand and Food and Agriculture Organization of the United Nations, Rome, Italy.

Subasinghe, R.P., S.E. McGladdery, and B. Hill. 2004. *Surveillance and Zoning for Aquatic Animal Diseases.* FAO Fisheries Technical Paper No. 451. Food and Agriculture Organization of the United Nations, Rome, Italy. 73 pp.

Ward, M. and T. Carpenter. 2000. Analysis of space-time clustering in veterinary epidemiology. *Preventive Veterinary Medicine* 43:225–237.

Appendix

Appendix: Mechanisms of surveillance (Adapted from Scudamore 2002)

Mechanism	Description	Advantages	Disadvantages	Comments	Relative cost
Outbreak investigation	Personnel with appropriate expertise and resources required to investigate outbreaks of unusual disease syndromes.	"Syndrome surveillance" provides a route for identifying novel conditions.	Depends on clear, agreed definitions of a "case" and an "outbreak" for the particular syndrome of interest and agreed "intervention levels." Depends on good relationship between industry and investigators, and, therefore, misses those sectors without this relationship.	Variety of observation points may trigger investigations.	Can be high if intervention levels not appropriate
Voluntary notification	Observation of disease is reported to responsible government agency either directly or through routinely reviewed publications or other sources. e.g., Unusual clinical syndrome.	Provides a route for new and unusual syndromes to be identified. Can be effective if farmers, fishermen, and others are motivated to report. Useful for recording unusual events of limited consequence.	Will miss cases due to under-reporting (poor sensitivity). Hard to define or measure the denominator, so trends cannot be evaluated. Indirectly reported disease events only captured by government surveillance program if information gathering structure exists.	Reports are received when the observed disease is recognized and the observer is aware of the route by which the report can be submitted. Can be improved by increasing awareness (e.g., by specific campaigns) and by offering financial incentives, but both increase cost.	Low

Compulsory notification	Legal obligation for observer to report specific disease events suspected to be of concern to responsible government agency. Such events have a legal definition. e.g., Notifiable diseases in different countries.	Good for syndromes that are easily recognized, particularly if awareness is raised. Requirement to notify is uniform across the country. Notification facilitates the swift implementation of investigation and control measures. Clinical notification enables action to be taken in respect of diseases that are not rapidly or routinely confirmed in a laboratory. Location details are supplied with notification, which may assist calculation of infection rates, and comparison of infections over time and geographic area.	Under-reporting is likely, unless training in awareness of clinical presentation and route of reporting is maintained among the appropriate people. The level of under-reporting of a particular disease is often biased; there are many reasons why a report may not be made, and these can be different for different areas or types of stakeholder interest. Reduced sensitivity for syndromes that resemble endemic disease syndromes. Events with non-specific signs may be missed (poor specificity). Adverse impact on stakeholder as a consequence of reporting may act as a disincentive and can increase under-reporting, e.g., where disease prevents export. Where it is not be possible to estimate population size, incidence or prevalence rates cannot be calculated.	Reports are received when the observed event is recognized or suspected of being "notifiable" and as being subject to statute, and the observer is aware of the route by which a report should be submitted. Can be improved with incentives such as compensation.	Low when prevalence is low

(*Continues*)

Appendix (*Continued*)

Mechanism	Description	Advantages	Disadvantages	Comments	Relative cost
Sentinel systems—primary and secondary information sources	Key observers are recruited to provide routine returns listing the type, number, and other specified details of specified events that are observed. Events of interest are defined and may differ in different periods of time. Sentinels can be primary sources, such as industry stakeholders, or secondary, such as aquatic animal health personnel.	Can be trained for the purpose, giving good specificity. Specialized and trained sentinels can provide sensitive and moderately specific estimates of level of defined events in the population of interest. Flexible. Once network recruited and established syndromes of interest and data to be collected can be varied in response to changing needs. Can provide data on common conditions that are not notifiable and for which laboratory diagnosis is not routine. An estimate of the population size under surveillance many be available so population-based rates can be calculated. If sentinel sites are representative, estimates can be generalized to a wider population. Additional information that enables interpretation to trends can be collected. Can monitor the reason for, and outcome of particular laboratory tests or other health event, so improved interpretation of other surveillance data.	Not useful for rare events, as sentinels usually cover a small proportion of the population under surveillance (because of costs). Can be difficult to recruit sentinels that are representative of the population of interest so results may be biased.	Observers are recruited appropriate to the event(s) to be surveyed for. Specificity can be improved by linking field observers with diagnostic laboratoriesTo be effective, contact must be maintained and regular feedback provided, so as to retain the commitment of.	Moderate to high

Sentinel systems—tertiary data sources	Contributed data (e.g., from diagnostic laboratories) includes number of diagnoses made for particular diseases with a variable amount of supporting information such as species affected, date of diagnosis, geographic location, specimen type etc. These can be collated to provide national statistics that can indicate long-term trends and the effects of interventions.	Efficient surveillance method for indicators that cannot be confirmed by primary or secondary data sources (e.g., diseases with non-specific clinical signs). Can be universal, involving all sources, with a broad range of indicators reported, so it is sensitive enough to detect rare but important changes at an early stage (e.g., emergence of new diseases). Can provide information on the relative morbidity due to particular indicators (e.g., causes of poor reproduction) and so guide the setting of priorities. Highly specific, where accredited and quality controlled data sources are used, so links between cases reported from different areas can be recognized. Provides a mechanism for identifying cases that can contribute to further study of priority diseases where more information is required. Data on some indicators are not routinely available by any other means.	Under-reporting is likely (as dependent on primary and secondary data sources for material), so it is impossible to calculate the total number of cases of disease. May not be universal. Distribution of contributing laboratories may not be comprehensive, leading to geographical "blind spots." Cases that are easily diagnosed at primary and secondary level will not contribute to the data, as no need to refer cases or diagnostic material. The frequency of diagnosis is biased by the rate at which cases or specimens are referred; if the same factors *affect all groups* (e.g., economic hardship), relative morbidities will still be valid. However, certain population or disease sub-groups may be affected to a greater or lesser degree (e.g., availability of a new vaccine). There is no tertiary diagnostic support for some diseases in some countries.	—	Variable, but usually moderate to high

(*Continues*)

Appendix (*Continued*)

Mechanism	Description	Advantages	Disadvantages	Comments	Relative cost
Structured surveys	A selected sample of the population of interest is surveyed for a particular disease(s) and other possible factors of interest.	The population of interest and the information needed can be defined. Provided a population list (sampling frame) exists, the data must be collected from a representative sample of the population so prevalence or incidence can be measured. The survey can be repeated over time to evaluate trends. A range of surveys can be carried out which are targeted at different populations to define the overall level and distribution of disease. Cost can be controlled by restricting the precision of the estimate.	Targeted, so can only give population estimates for diseases and factors that are specified in the study design. Cannot usually respond to new information, or diseases that are new or unexpected. Differences in diagnostic methods or changes over time can limit the comparability of surveys that set out to measure the same thing. Can have problems with non-participation. Baseline data sets may be incomplete or unavailable. Can be very expensive if sample sizes are large and access to remote sub-populations difficult.	Small sample size surveys can give useful results provided the disease or syndrome of interest is not rare. Cost depends on disease characteristics and precision required.	Variable, but usually moderate to high
Census	Measurement of an indicator in all members of a defined population. e.g., testing of all shrimp broodstock for WSD.	All members of the defined population contribute information so true prevalence or incidence can be measured.	Requires a mechanism for identifying all members of the population to be counted. Expensive.	—	High

Chapter 10

Biosecurity at the Farm Level—How to Create a State of Mind

Paul Hardy-Smith

Abstract

Creating biosecurity awareness is about creating a state of mind. This chapter discusses why having biosecurity "aware" farm managers and farm workers can significantly minimize risk in an aquaculture facility and how to develop this "awareness" at the farm level. Examples are used to highlight the value of having aware staff and also the consequences of not having such staff. Seven key steps that can be used to help create such a state of mind and biosecurity awareness at the farm level are then discussed.

Introduction

Biosecurity is a relatively new and evolving concept. For the Food and Agricultural Organization of the United Nations (FAO), biosecurity broadly describes the process and objective of managing biological risks associated with food and agriculture in a holistic manner (FAO 2003). To the farmer, concepts are not useful or practical until they result in something real, the overall objective being to ensure economic viability and profitability of the enterprise.

The understanding of biosecurity varies considerably at the farm level. So too does the understanding of what actions are required to achieve adequate "biosecurity." To some, biosecurity is simply about having barriers in place that are designed to ensure pathogen exclusion from a farm site. One of the most common and arguably least effective manifestations of this understanding is epitomized by the provision of footbaths at one or more of the entrances to a farm site. While their usefulness for ensuring pathogen exclusion is highly debatable (especially when disinfectant solutions are not refreshed on a regular basis), they are often justified merely due to their presence in maintaining "awareness" in farm staff and visitors. It is questionable how effective the "awareness" created in this way is. Even more questionable is the effectiveness or usefulness of such "barriers" in aquaculture operations where there is little opportunity to control the movement of potential pathogens between the

---

Paul Hardy-Smith, E-mail: info@panaquatic.com

cultured aquatic animals and the environment. One such example is the farming of aquatic animals in floating netpens at sea.

Farm staff are the eyes and ears of the operation. It takes time, however, to create staff in biosecurity awareness that will help to ensure the economic viability and profitability of the enterprise. It is about creating a state of mind in staff so that they are alert at all times to any possible threat that could affect the health and well-being of the aquatic animals under their care. This chapter discusses two examples that show the importance of having biosecurity aware staff and the consequences of having unaware staff. It then discusses a seven-step process that is designed to ensure a high level of awareness in farm staff, irrespective of the size of the farm.

Importance of biosecurity "awareness"

The following two examples indicate the importance of biosecurity awareness, and more particularly, awareness in the farm staff themselves.

Example 1: Consequences of a lack of awareness

Approximately 100,000 Atlantic salmon (*Salmo salar*) smolts (i.e., salmon that have undergone a morphological and physiological change in preparation for moving from the freshwater environment to the saltwater environment) were being transported in a well-boat. Saltwater from the surrounding waters was continually pumped through the wells in the boat during the journey to the sea site. The journey lasted 12 hours and the chosen route deliberately avoided other fish farming areas.

The company had its own technician on the boat, monitoring the health and well-being of the fish during the journey. The technician was relatively new to the company, had little training in fish health, and his enthusiasm for his work was questionable.

About half way through the journey, the technician noticed another boat releasing a dark material into the channel through which the well boat was sailing. The technician knew the boat was involved in harvesting farmed salmon and thought that the material being released was dirty bilge water. As the well-boat, however, approached the plume, the technician realized the harvest boat was pumping out bloodwater. The well-boat sailed through the plume of bloodwater, and the wells of the boat holding the fish quickly darkened as the bloodwater was pumped through the fish on board.

The technician did not know that the harvest boat had just finished offloading harvested fish taken from a site that was undergoing a serious disease outbreak. The harvest boat was required to disinfect the bloodwater prior to release, but the effectiveness of the disinfection procedure used had not been fully evaluated.

The technician had heard of there being some disease concerns in the industry, but was more concerned with getting the trip over and getting home. As the fish did not appear to be suffering while the darker water was circulating through the holds, no action was taken and no one was notified about the incident.

The well-boat motored for another 6 hours before arriving at the sea site and offloading the fish. Initially, the fish appeared healthy. However, 2 weeks later, some of the fish began showing clinical signs of disease. Four weeks later, more than half the fish from that trip had died and most of the other fish on the site were starting to show signs of disease. In all, more than 80% of the fish died on the site.

The technician's lack of biosecurity awareness and resultant lack of action cost the company many thousands of dollars.

Example 2: The value of awareness

Fish on a large fish farm were suffering from low-grade mortality due to a bacterial disease. This disease caused significant hemorrhaging (bleeding) in the fish. The farm manager had been well trained in all aspects of fish health and was very proud of the fish on his site and of the site itself. He was in constant communication with the company veterinarian, discussing what was happening in the industry with respect to disease, disease outbreaks, and fish health issues in general. The company veterinarian, together with the other farm managers in the company, had developed a classification system for fish mortalities and had done a lot of fish health training on the farm site. The classification system required that a certain percentage of the dead fish were opened up on site so that an examination of the internal organs could be made. Prior to this, only an external examination was made of dead fish.

One day, when opening up some of the dead fish that had been collected from one of the pens, the manager noted a difference in the pattern of internal hemorrhaging in the fish. In the fish dying from the bacterial disease, the hemorrhaging had been confined to the swim bladder and was usually scattered diffusely throughout the gut cavity and sometimes on the surface of internal organs such as the liver (Fig. 10.1). In the fish he had opened in front of him, the hemorrhaging was concentrated in the upper areas of the front of the gut cavity. The farm manager had also noticed far more blood tinged fluid around the internal organs when he had opened the fish (Fig. 10.2).

The change was subtle, but the farm manager was aware that the pattern of hemorrhage in disease outbreaks due to a viral disease was different. He rang the company

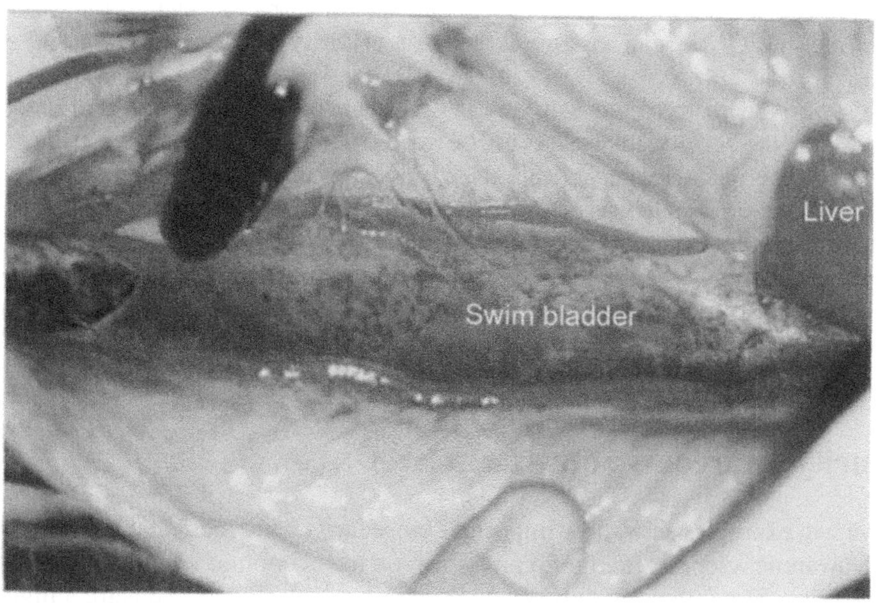

Fig. 10.1 Fish that had died of bacterial disease. Note hemorrhage on the swim bladder.

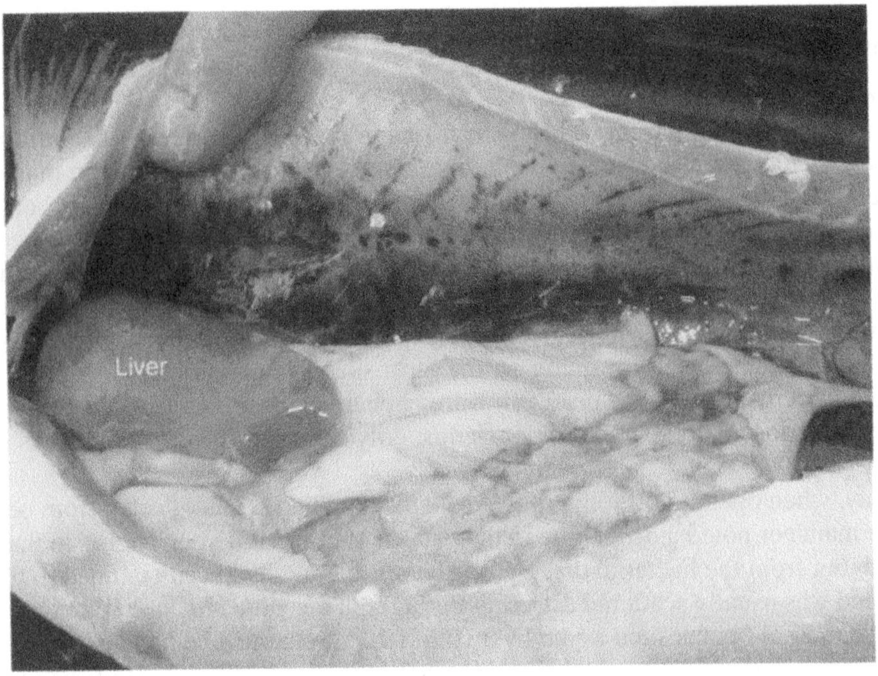

Fig. 10.2 Fish with different patterns of hemorrhage. Note significant hemorrhage in the upper part of gut cavity above liver.

veterinarian to discuss his finding. The company veterinarian was extremely concerned and instructed the manager to place the fish into a sealed plastic bag. After informing the General Manager (GM) of the company about his concerns, he visited the farm site. In the meantime, the GM began investigating the feasibility of harvesting the site ahead of schedule.

Samples were taken from the fish, and it was confirmed that the fish had died of viral infection. While the bacterial disease could be treated with antibiotics, the viral disease could not. Industry experience suggested that the virus had the potential to cause mortalities in excess of 50%, hence the site was harvested at an increased rate ahead of schedule to remove the valuable fish from the water before they succumbed to disease.

Biosecurity awareness of the farm manager and having a system to classify mortalities that improved the ability of farm staff to identify different disease signs saved the company many thousands of dollars.

Biosecurity awareness at the farm level

The above two examples show how important biosecurity awareness at the farm level is and how such awareness, or lack thereof, can impact on the economic viability and profitability of an enterprise. The following outlines a process that is designed to ensure a high level of awareness in farm staff, irrespective of the size of the farm.

Start with the right people

Sometimes, one has to make do with what one has, but, if possible, employing people who are keen, willing to learn, and motivated can significantly help the process. Disgruntled employees can seriously jeopardize the process.

Instill a sense of pride in what farm staff do and in the venture/company

Farm staff who are proud of their farm and proud of the company they work for are far more willing to do what it takes to protect the health of the aquatic animals they are farming than unhappy or disgruntled staff. Creating this sense of pride and caring for employees will pay dividends in the process. This is often not easy, requiring the creation of a positive company or enterprise culture in which staff are made to feel important and valued.

Train farm staff in the skills of fish health (including an understanding of the concept of biosecurity)

Education is at the heart of creating biosecurity awareness. It instills in the farm staff an understanding of potential sources of health risks and importantly, how to maintain optimum health in the aquatic animals under their care. Maintaining optimum health is a cornerstone of biosecurity; having healthy stock decreases the overall risk of disease. Having farm staff take training courses at a college or institution can expedite the teaching process, but it must go further than this. Farm staff need to understand how the training relates to their own farm and make sure a significant portion of this learning is farm based. Applied training at the farm site itself will ensure this understanding.

Let farm staff improve on what they have been taught, i.e., give them some ownership of the process

It is important to have standard operating procedures (SOPs) and systems in place to minimize the fish health risks on a farm. The implementation of such systems and procedures can help ensure consistency throughout different operations within a company or enterprise and is necessary and worthwhile. Enrollment of the farm staff themselves, however, in the development and creation of these SOPs and systems is sometimes overlooked. Allowing them to contribute encourages ownership and increased commitment and can make a significant contribution to the effectiveness of the farm or organization.

Ensure farm staff use the skills they have been taught to benefit the enterprise

A good example is the recording of mortalities. Motivated farm staff want to learn about what they are growing. From an operations perspective, it is extremely useful to have staff who are knowledgeable about what a "normal" fish/crustacean/mollusc looks like, both inside and out, and to be able to identify what does *not* look normal. A mortality recording system can be designed so that it encourages farm staff to look at mortalities and categorize their causes. This greatly assists in record keeping and aquatic animal health monitoring, and also maintains and improves the farm staff's skills in early recognition of disease.

Databases that are custom designed for documenting mortality numbers and rates and for classifying mortalities based on what the farmer is seeing (e.g., "internal swelling," "skin/fin erosion") are useful tools in maintaining biosecurity awareness at the farm level. Even small enterprises can benefit by adopting such databases, especially if substantial growth of the enterprise is expected.

Keep staff up-to-date with industry knowledge

There is often a failure of top management to ensure farm staff are kept informed of important health developments in their own industry. For example, knowledge that there has been a fish health problem on a neighboring farm or in the local area is critical information for the farm staff, especially if there is any indication that the cause of the problem may be infectious. Fortunately, it is quite common for farmers from different farms and companies to talk among themselves, but this "grapevine" should not be relied on as a substitute for factual information being provided by the top management in a timely manner.

Maintain good communication channels

It is absolutely critical to encourage biosecurity awareness, and minimize risk for the enterprise. Farm staff like to talk about what they are doing; and to varying degrees, they are the eyes and ears of the enterprise. They are constantly observing the fish or other cultured species and what is happening in and around their farm. They often have concerns. Being able to discuss such concerns may assist in the early identification of potential biosecurity problems, and allow prompt action to be taken to ensure the problems are dealt with so as to have minimal impact on the enterprise.

Importantly, it also helps if the farm staff can discuss such concerns at an informal level with a professional who is knowledgeable on aquatic animal health and biosecurity and whom they trust and respect. Such a relationship can take time to develop but is well worth the effort.

Conclusion

Biosecurity awareness at the farm level is not simply about having footbaths at the entrance to a facility. Biosecurity awareness is the creation of a state of mind in farm staff such that there is constant vigilance at the farm level, on fish health issues that may impact the profitability and sustainability of the enterprise. It is not created overnight, but requires effort and resources. Finally, though, the cost benefit associated with that effort will be positive and significant.

References

FAO (Food and Agricultural Organization of the United Nations). 2003. *Committee on Agriculture Seventeenth Session Rome*, 31 March–4 April 2003, Biosecurity in Food and Agriculture. Item 9 of the Provisional Agenda. On-line version, http://www.fao.org/DOCREP/MEETING/006/Y8453E.HTM#P35_2595

Chapter 11

Elements of an Aquatic Animal Health Program—Infectious Hematopoietic Necrosis in Farmed Atlantic Salmon in British Columbia

Grace A. Karreman

Abstract

Infectious hematopoietic necrosis (IHN) has been a devastating disease of farmed Atlantic salmon (*Salmo salar* L.) in British Columbia (BC), Canada, with two epizootics occurring in the past 12 years. This disease has been documented in Pacific salmon (*Oncorhynchus* spp.) and was most likely introduced from the wild. In the 2001–2003 epizootic, one-third to one-half of the active production sites were affected. Industry undertook voluntary depopulation and other measures to control the outbreak.

Saksida (2003, personal communication) did a review and analysis of potential risk factors related to introduction and spread of the disease in the most recent epizootic. Industry made changes in husbandry practices including: development of management protocols in conjunction with the British Columbia Ministry of Agriculture, Food and Fisheries (BC MAFF), changes to methods of transporting fish, changes to harvesting operations, and disinfection of processing plant discharge. Efforts are underway to validate a reverse transcription polymerase chain reaction for rapid detection and to develop an effective IHN vaccine.

Regulatory changes included mandatory Fish Health Plans in which operators must document how they meet required fish health practices. British Columbia MAFF does quarterly surveillance sampling on randomly selected sites and checks farm records and for submissions to a third-party fish health database.

Both the province and the federal governments have supported research efforts directed at disease management and effective biosecurity. The most significant missing component, however, remains a lack of knowledge of the disease/infection status of wild fish and the dynamics of disease transmission between wild and farmed fish. The dynamics of disease transmission in the aquatic medium are poorly understood. Improved biosecurity with respect to this disease will require a multi-tiered, multiple stakeholder approach based on sound aquatic animal health research and management practices.

Grace A. Karreman, E-mail: karreman@shaw.ca

Introduction

Aquatic animal biosecurity must involve the competent application of biosecurity concepts and experiences from terrestrial species to the aquatic situation. A consistent definition of "aquatic biosecurity," however, at the farm, regional, and national level has not yet been formulated. Aquatic biosecurity concerns depart from their terrestrial counterparts due to the disproportionately large influence of the aquatic environment. The aquatic environment acts both as an effective medium for infectious pathogen/disease transmission and home to species whose ecology and role in disease transfer is poorly if at all understood.

A practical approach at the farm level is the exclusion of pathogens, which when presented with a favorable combination of environment and host, could cause serious disease outbreaks on a site. A recent example is infectious hematopoietic necrosis (IHN), an emerging viral disease that caused high mortality rates in farmed Atlantic salmon (*Salmo salar* L.) at marine netpen sites in British Columbia. In 1992–1996 and 2001–2003, IHN occurred at epidemic levels at Atlantic salmon farms. While this disease had been documented in Pacific salmon (*Oncorhynchus* spp.) for decades preceding the development of IHN among commercial aquaculture operations, in BC it was unique in that it affected salmon at marine farm sites, particularly Atlantic salmon.

The BC salmon farming industry, with assistance from provincial veterinary fish health authorities, had to develop control measures for this disease, including detailed biosecurity protocols, to survive. A major component of developing the control measures was a veterinary study commissioned by the BC Ministry of Agriculture, Food and Fisheries (BC MAFF) to investigate the descriptive epidemiology of the most recent outbreak, evaluate the potential risk factors for the disease, and make recommendations for its management. This chapter provides a brief summary of a full report from a study undertaken to evaluate the potential risk factors associated with the disease at the farm level and the biosecurity measures that were recommended, implemented, or both, as a result of the study.

Collaboration between the industry and the provincial government in part helped to bring the disease under control. "Big picture" aquatic biosecurity in BC, however, still must address significant gaps in knowledge about wild populations that could harbor or act as reservoirs for the disease.

The 2001 IHN outbreak

Description

Saksida reviewed the 2001–2003 IHN epizootic in BC (Saksida 2003). During that period, IHN virus (IHNV) was detected on 36 Atlantic salmon sites located in five of the seven geographic farming regions.

In affected farms, mortality rates averaged from 40% to 70%, with the smallest fish most affected. The outbreak was brought under control in 23 months (Saksida 2003). Affected companies voluntarily depopulated seven sites, tightened biosecurity procedures as a control measure, or took both courses of action. Nevertheless, 12 million fish died or were culled as a result of the outbreak, resulting in millions of dollars lost in direct and indirect costs, most if not all of which were borne by the individual companies (Saksida personal communication).

IHNV

The index case was diagnosed in late summer. Two separate viral isolates were seen: one on the east coast of Vancouver Island in August 2001 and an other on the west coast the following March, each representing an independent introduction of IHNV into farmed salmon (Saksida 2003). Both isolates are similar to the endemic forms commonly found in the region.

Risk factors

Subsequent to the first epizootic (1992–1996), husbandry practices were modified, including single year class stocking at sites, use of an autogenous vaccine for prevention, improved fish health monitoring, and increased awareness of IHNV at the sites (Saksida personal communication).

As part of the BC MAFF study during the 2001–2003 epizootic, Saksida (2003) interviewed all companies with affected sites and developed a list of possible risk factors and underlying hypotheses associated with increased risk of IHN in Atlantic salmon. Six factors were identified that may have contributed to horizontal transmission in seawater.

- Returning wild sockeye salmon (*Oncorhynchus nerka*) may have accounted for the index case. While the disease transmission dynamics between farmed and wild fish are unknown, experiments have shown that Atlantic salmon could be infected when cohabiting with infected salmon (Traxler et al. 1993).
- The likely route of transmission within a marine site was waterborne. In addition, given tidal circulation patterns in BC, an affected site could also provide the source for infection to the sites "downstream" from the first site.
- IHNV has been documented in other species that may have acted as carriers of IHNV in the outbreak, e.g., herring in the wild and in experimental challenge studies, in Chinook salmon and in shiner perch (*Cymatogaster aggregata*) and tubesnout (*Aulorhynchus flavidus*) (Kent et al. 1998; Kocan et al. 1997; Traxler et al. 1998; St-Hilaire et al. 2001; Traxler and Richard 1996). The disease transmission dynamics are unknown, but some of these species were observed near fish farms during the epizootic.
- The risk of spreading IHN by moving Atlantic salmon within an infected area was very high, particularly if tow pens were used. The same may have been true for converted fish boats/packers due to their inability to completely seal water intakes or hatches.
- Shared equipment or movement of multi-use vessels may have contributed to spread of the infection, due to lack of effective disinfection by failure to move all infected organic material or water.
- Although almost all harvest sites adhered to the disinfection protocol for blood water and processing water (see BC MAFF 2004c), disinfection efficacy may have been compromised by the level of organic material and the reduced effectiveness of chlorine in seawater (Torgersen and Hastein 1995).

Saksida (2003) identified three additional potential factors.

1. Because the diagnosis was confirmed by viral culture, which is time-intensive, there was an average lag time of 15.7 days between suspicion and confirmation of the diagnosis. Due to costs associated with implementation of increased biosecurity, appropriate measures were often not undertaken until after the diagnosis was confirmed.
2. The data implied that several stressors, such as poor water quality (e.g., low dissolved oxygen levels, plankton blooms), concurrent disease, and/or husbandry factors, such as fish handling, may have been present prior to the onset of IHN.
3. There was no effective vaccine. Variable protection was seen in fish vaccinated with a commercially manufactured autogenous product prior to the outbreak.

Toward the future

Saksida (2003) made more than 40 recommendations regarding reducing the risk of contracting IHN, spreading IHN, or both. Chief among these were to conduct research into wild fish health status and transmission dynamics between wild and farmed fish, to establish management zones, to implement measures for managing a confirmed positive site, to equip vessels properly for transporting fish, to develop industry-wide protocols for communications and standardized biosecurity protocols for suppliers and visitors as well as sites, to develop and validate a test for early detection of IHNV, and to develop an effective vaccine.

Commercial companies had already responded to the disease on a site-by-site basis (Saksida personal communication). All sites established isolation protocols when a diagnosis of IHN was made. The rate of mortality removal was increased, either through dramatically increased rates of mortality dives during the initial high mortality periods, or by instituting secondary non-diving recovery systems on the farms, such as "uplift" and "mort ring" systems. On-site dive protocols were changed in some companies so that each site had its own dive gear rather than using a dive team that moved from site to site with potentially insufficient disinfection between sites.

Certain companies altered their harvesting protocol so that fish were killed only by stunning (by a percussive blow to the head) on site, and then shipped unbled to the processing plant to alleviate concerns about the ability to fully contain the blood water on-site. Another company worked on developing closed, disinfected recirculating water systems on dedicated vessels for transporting live fish.

Some companies made specific biosecurity protocols a condition of contract for their suppliers, particularly those such as feed and other services that were known to have contact with growing sites located outside the company.

Finally, there was cooperation between the industry and government. Even though IHN is not a listed reportable disease in BC, all of the companies kept the provincial and the federal government agencies informed of positive results. The companies, working in conjunction with BC MAFF, suggested practices to minimize risks beyond those listed in the BCSFA code of practices. These included protocols for isolation of affected sites, handling fish on affected sites or within a positive zone, disinfection protocols, and processing/harvesting of infected fish (BC MAFF 2004c).

Short-term outcome

The effectiveness of these and many other activities cannot be measured until there is another introduction of the virus, should it occur. The most recent epizootic, however, was brought under control in 23 months, with no further outbreaks having been reported since June 2003. When revised protocols were instituted, including biosecurity awareness by fish plant operators, no new outbreaks were seen in recently entered smolts transported past the fish plant that might have been involved with inadvertent disease transfer. By the end of 2003, most plants that process farmed salmon had set up treatment facilities to successfully disinfect harvest by-products.

Next steps

The industry has acknowledged the need to evaluate and improve other practices related to site biosecurity (including boat traffic monitoring), fish movement practices, disinfection protocols for multi-farm equipment, such as fouled barges and nets, contingency plans for removing large numbers of mortalities/culls, and standard operating procedures for supplier vessels. The need to remove diseased populations quickly has also been recognized. A new set of rules needs to be established, particularly for the index case. Cooperation of all of the potentially affected companies is essential, particularly with regard to cost sharing and insurance arrangements (Saksida personal communication).

A reliable, validated early detection technique is essential for managing the disease. The conflict between the shortest time from apparent exposure to the virus to the appearance of clinical disease of 7 days, and the average lag time between suspicion and confirmation of an infection of 15.7 days, continues to be a risk. There is a reverse transcription polymerase chain reaction (RT-PCR) test that can be used directly on fish tissue and could supply results in less than 2 days. This technique, while promising, has not yet been validated and thus cannot be considered the definitive diagnostic test for IHN. Also, there is concern that this technique cannot distinguish fish that had been vaccinated against IHNV from fish that are infected with the virus, possibly leading to false-positive results. Proper validation and standardization of this protocol could make it a valuable tool in the future, but development and/or evaluation of method other than viral culture or PCR for early detection and diagnosis of IHNV should be a priority.

Both epidemiological and economical considerations make IHNV an excellent candidate for a vaccine. At present, there are no effective IHN viral vaccines commercially available. Newer technologies, however, are being investigated.

While it is still not proven that horizontal transfer in seawater from returning Pacific species such as sockeye has occurred, it may be necessary to provide alternate stocking strategies/timing for channels in which these returning wild stocks are known to migrate and in which the disease has previously been seen. Similarly, farming Pacific species on the same site or in the same area as Atlantic species should be avoided, and methods for minimizing contact with other, non-migratory finfish that may be hosts or carriers for IHNV should be investigated.

Other preventative or mitigative strategies may need to involve additional stakeholders in the marine resource. For example, IHN is also a common disease in wild salmonids in BC, such as sockeye, and the majority of the processing plants that handle wild fish still do not treat their process water prior to discharge. Untreated effluent from these facilities could still pose a substantial risk to the farmed fish population.

Regulatory role

In part due to the IHN outbreaks, the provincial government (through BC MAFF) imposed fish health regulations as a condition of license for all aquaculture operators in the province. Foremost among these regulatory requirements were the Fish Health Management Plans, a set of required fish health practices for all culture facilities, developed with input from industry. These plans became mandatory in the spring of 2004.

Each operator has to detail how he or she would meet the required practices. Each site or company must have a relationship with a veterinarian (or fish health professional if there is no veterinarian), conduct routine monitoring of fish health, outbreak management and investigation, report monthly mortality information and fish health events requiring intervention to a third-party central database, and report major outbreaks including IHN to BC MAFF. The Fish Health Management Plan of each operator must also detail how a disease outbreak (e.g., IHN) would be handled at those sites and include details on mass mortality management as well as isolation, site biosecurity, reporting, and attaining a positive diagnosis. Fish Health Management Plans must be kept on file, be accessible, and be approved by a BC MAFF Fish Health Veterinarian (BC MAFF 2004d).

British Columbia MAFF also monitors fish health activity on the sites on a routine basis. Each quarter, 30 operational sites (or 25% of active sites, whichever number is greater) are randomly selected by the Fish Health Auditing and Surveillance Program according to species and geographic area for sampling and surveillance (BC MAFF 2004a). The sampling is done the same day as the site mortality dive. Thirty fish are randomly selected from all pens for a full health workup. The program has been in operation since 2001, and the results are maintained in a BC MAFF database.

In addition to site sampling and surveillance, BC MAFF asks for recent history of disease or unexplained losses, and may also ask for records of the mortality and the fish health event data that have been submitted to the third-party central database. This second database maintained by the BC Salmon Farmers Association holds the individual disease incidence data from each site, and reports quarterly on an aggregate basis using the same species and geographic criteria defined for the surveillance program (BC MAFF 2004b). This public–private partnership allows information to be submitted on a confidential basis, but the company submitting the information is also subject to on-site verification so that the information is correct. Figure 11.1 shows the relationship of each component.

Research needs

Significant commitment to applied research is required if the disease management and biosecurity issues concerning IHN in Atlantic salmon in BC are to be addressed. In addition to the risk factor study, BC MAFF, with support from Fisheries and Oceans Canada (DFO) and private sector suppliers sponsored an IHN research workshop in January 2003. Researchers with diverse specialties addressed research and management needs. A White Paper (Karreman and Stephen 2003) summarizing the proceedings and recommendations

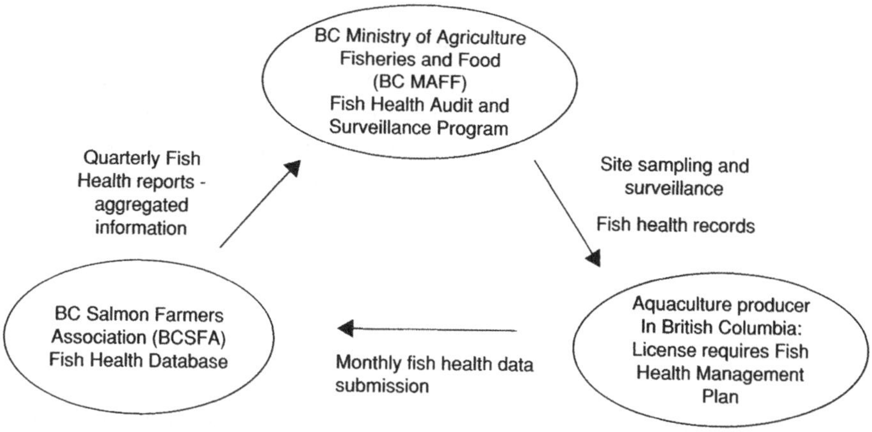

Fig. 11.1 Relationship of major fish health components in British Columbia.

of the workshop supported the research recommendations by Saksida (2003). It also pointed out the significant gaps in diagnostic and research capacity in BC, as well as in coordination and extension. Participants agreed that urgent research was required for:

1. field validation of rapid detection techniques, particularly PCR;
2. investigation into viral source, spread, and transmission by, e.g.,
   - identifying the routes of viral movement;
   - characterizing water currents around farms to assist in development of biologically sensible quarantine or exclusion zones;
   - identifying sources and environmental sinks of IHNV—specifically, wild fish, sea lice, biofouling (nets and boats), plankton, sediments, benthos (including shellfish), and fecal material;
   - identifying spatial and temporal patterns of viral shedding;
   - developing vaccines; and
   - conducting epidemiological studies, including
     a. conducting an observational study to quantify risk of IHN mortality at cage and site level, and
     b. Conducting case-control studies of affected and unaffected farms.

Health research in wild fish

British Columbia MAFF has subsequently helped to support several of the above research projects. The major (largely) unaddressed biosecurity and management component, however, is the role of wild fish in the index case and possible spread between sites. This involves both knowledge of the health status of those animals, e.g., are they reservoirs for the disease, as well as the dynamics of disease transmission between wild and farmed populations. A systematic surveillance effort will be required to address these issues, complemented by support for scientific investigations into the areas listed above. There has been some collaborative work between the industry, the province, and the DFO on laboratory investigations. Other than snapshot surveys (Kent et. al. 1998), however, and some targeted or convenience sampling (DFO 2004), there has been no systematic sampling effort for health status in wild salmonid stocks in general and for IHN in particular. Wild fish are a federal jurisdiction under the Fisheries Act (Canada), and significant federal support and epidemiological expertise will be required to set up a sound wild fish health research and surveillance program. It is hoped that efforts like the newly initiated National Aquatic Animal Health Plan will take on this responsibility and thereby complement the significant efforts already undertaken by the provincial government and the industry for health in farmed fish.

Summary

Infectious Hematopoietic Necrosis has been a devastating disease of farmed Atlantic salmon in BC, with two epizootics occurring in the last 12 years. This disease has been documented in Pacific salmon for decades preceding the development of commercial aquaculture and was most likely introduced from the wild. In the 2001–2003 epizootic, one-third to one-half of the active production sites were affected. Mortality rates varied from 40% to 70% and approximately 12 million farmed fish were affected. Industry undertook voluntary depopulation and other measures to control the outbreak.

Saksida (2003) did a review and analysis of potential risk factors related to introduction and spread of the disease in the most recent epizootic. Industry made changes in husbandry practices, including development of management protocols in conjunction with BC MAFF, changes to methods of transporting fish including vessels, changes to harvesting operations on-site, and disinfection of processing plant discharge. Further improvements need to be made; however, efforts are underway to validate an RT-PCR for rapid detection and to develop an effective IHN vaccine.

Regulatory changes included Fish Health Plans, which became a mandatory component of a BC aquaculture operator's license in the spring of 2003. Operators must document how they meet required fish health practices including health monitoring, disease detection and response, and reporting to BC MAFF and to a third-party central database. BC MAFF does quarterly surveillance sampling on randomly selected sites and checks farm records and for submissions to the third-party database.

Research needs to support disease management and effective biosecurity were documented by the risk factor study as well as an IHN research workshop in 2003. Both the province and the federal governments have supported research efforts directed at the priority areas. The most significant missing component, however, remains a lack of knowledge of the disease or infection status of wild fish and the dynamics of disease transmission between wild and farmed fish. Wild fish are under federal jurisdiction in Canada. Federal support, potentially through the recently initiated National Aquatic Animal Health Program, will be required to address surveillance and research of wild fish.

In general, and specifically for IHN, the dynamics of disease transmission in the aquatic medium are poorly understood. Knowledge will only come through quality aquatic health management research and practical, on-site aquatic animal health experience. Improved biosecurity with respect to this disease will require a multi-tiered, multiple stakeholder approach based on sound aquatic animal health research and management practices.

References

BC MAFF (British Columbia Ministry of Agriculture, Food and Fisheries). 2004a. *Fish Health Auditing and Surveillance Program (FHASP)*. British Columbia Ministry of Agriculture, Food and Fisheries, Victoria, British Columbia, Canada. On-line, http://www.agf.gov.bc.ca/fisheries/health/IHNV_Isolation_Control_Procedures.pdf.

BC MAFF (British Columbia Ministry of Agriculture, Food and Fisheries). 2004b. *BC Salmon Farmers Association Fish Health Database*. British Columbia Ministry of Agriculture, Food and Fisheries, Victoria, British Columbia, Canada. On-line, http://www.agf.gov.bc.ca/fisheries/health/bcsfa_database.htm.

BC MAFF (British Columbia Ministry of Agriculture, Food and Fisheries). 2004c. *Biosecurity Procedures for IHNV Positive Farm Sites*. British Columbia Ministry of Agriculture, Food and Fisheries, Victoria, British Columbia, Canada. On line, http://www.agf.gov.bc.ca/fisheries/health/IHNV_Isolation_Control_Procedures.pdf.

BC MAFF (British Columbia Ministry of Agriculture, Food and Fisheries). 2004d. *Fish Health Management Plan*. British Columbia Ministry of Agriculture, Food and Fisheries, Victoria, British Columbia, Canada. On line, http://www.agf.gov.bc.ca/fisheries/health/fish%5Fhealth%5Fmanagement%5Fplan.htm#Template.

DFO (Fisheries and Oceans Canada). 2004. *Pacific Region fish health database*. Fisheries and Oceans Canada, Ottawa, Ontario, Canada. On-line, http://www.pac.dfo-mpo.gc.ca.

Karreman, G.A. and C. Stephen. 2003. *White Paper: Infectious Hematopoietic Necrosis—Review and Consideration of a Workshop on IHN Research and Management Needs*. Prepared for Science Council of British Columbia and British Columbia Ministry of Agriculture, Food and Fisheries.

Kent, M.L., G.S. Traxler, D. Kieser, J. Richard, S.C. Dawe, R.W. Shaw, G. Prosperi-Porta, J. Ketcheson, and T.P.T. Evelyn. 1998. Survey of salmonid pathogens in ocean-caught fishes in British Columbia, Canada. *Journal of Aquatic Animal Health* 10:211–219.

Kocan, R., M. Bradley, N. Elder, T. Meyers, W. Bratts, and J. Winton. 1997. North American strain of viral hemorrhagic septicemia virus is highly pathogenic for laboratory-reared Pacific herring. *Journal of Aquatic Animal Health* 9:279–290.

Saksida, S. 2003. *Investigation of the 2001–2003 IHN Epizootic in Farmed Atlantic Salmon in British Columbia*. British Columbia Ministry of Agriculture, Food and Fisheries, Victoria, British Columbia, Canada. On line, http://www.agf.gov.bc.ca/fisheries/health/IHNV_report_2003.pdf.

St-Hilaire, S., C. Ribble, G. Traxler, T. Davies, and M.L. Kent. 2001. Evidence for a carrier state of infectious hematopoietic necrosis virus in chinook salmon *Oncorhynchus tshawytacha*. *Diseases of Aquatic Organisms* 46:173–179.

Torgersen, Y. and T. Hastein. 1995. Disinfection in Aquaculture. Scientific and technical review. *Office International des Epizooties* 14(2):419–434.

Traxler, G.S. and J. Richard. 1996. First detection of infectious hematopoietic necrosis virus in marine fishes. *Fish Health Section/American Fisheries Society Newsletter* 24:7.

Traxler, G.S., J.R. Roome, and M.L. Kent. 1993. Transmission of infectious hematopoietic necrosis virus in seawater. *Diseases of Aquatic Organisms* 16:111–114.

Traxler, G.S., M.L. Kent, and T.T. Poppe. 1998. Viral diseases. *in* Kent, M.L. and T.T. Poppe, editors. *Diseases of Seawater Netpen-Reared Salmonid Fishes*. Fisheries and Oceans, Canada, Ottawa, Ontario, Canada. 138 pp.

References

Chapter 12

A Preliminary Investigation of the Relationship between Infected Cage Removal Speed and Resultant Spread of Infectious Salmon Anemia on Atlantic Salmon Farms in Maine, U.S.A., and New Brunswick, Canada

Lori Gustafson, Stephen Ellis, Leighanne Hawkins, Mark Moore, Teresa Robinson, and Dan MacPhee

Abstract

Early removal of infected cages is considered to be an important step in the management of infectious salmon anemia(ISA). However, the costly depopulation of large numbers of fish can be difficult to motivate, especially prior to obvious clinical manifestations of disease. The authors conducted a retrospective evaluation of removal practices among Maine and New Brunswick farms that were (a) clients of Maritime Veterinary Services, (b) willing to share comprehensive data, and (c) diagnosed with ISA virus (ISAV) infection during a particular production cycle. Empirical evaluation of veterinary records from the nine farms meeting these inclusion criteria suggests a protective relationship between speedy removals of ISAV-infected cages and disease spread to other cages on a site. Shorter intervals between diagnosis and depopulation of index cages corresponded with greater cumulative proportions of non-infected cages 2, 3, and 4 months post-diagnosis ($p < 0.05$). The same dataset suggests a tendency (though not statistically significant) toward longer respites between diagnoses of index and secondary cages at sites practicing early removal. This retrospective study suggests that early removal of ISAV-infected cages may limit the extent of spread of ISAV throughout an infected site.

Lori Gustafson, corresponding author. E-mail: lori.l.gustafson@aphis.usda.gov

Introduction

Infectious salmon anemia (ISA) is an infectious disease of salmonids, caused by a virus in the Orthomyxoviridae family (Mjaaland et al. 1997; Krossoy et al. 1999) that often leads to extensive morbidity and mortality on affected farms (Thorud and Djupvik 1988; Byrne et al. 1998). Since its introduction to New Brunswick in 1996 (Mullins et al. 1998; Lovely et al. 1999) and Maine in 2001 (Bouchard et al. 2001), the disease has been difficult to control. Early diagnosis of ISA virus (ISAV) infection is based on a combination of assessments derived from a series of laboratory tests (indirect fluorescent antibody technique [IFAT], reverse transcription polymerase chain reaction [RT-PCR], and cell culture), clinical observations of moribund fish, cage mortality rates, and observed gross pathology (USDA APHIS Veterinary Services 2002; NBDAFA 2004).

Efforts to control ISA center on biosecurity and biocontainment (USDA APHIS Veterinary Services 2002; NBDAFA 2004). Biosecurity, preventing pathogen *introduction* to clean sites, and biocontainment, preventing pathogen *dispersal* from infected sites, go hand-in-hand. Biosecurity practices include routine cleaning and disinfection of vessels, equipment, and gear, the use of site-specific crews and equipment, restricted movements of vessels, single year class zoning, and a pre-stocking fallow period to limit the crossover of virus and/or vectors (e.g., sea lice *Lepeophtheirus salmonis*) from 1 year class to the next. Biocontainment, in contrast, hinges on the early identification and removal of infectious material and vector control: frequent dives to remove any dead/dying fish from cages; integrated pest management programs including aggressive sea lice monitoring; monthly site inspections by accredited veterinarians; routine submission of moribund fish for diagnostic testing; and depopulation of infected cages while the prevalence of ISA in the cage is still low. Without effective biocontainment, the job of prevention is extremely difficult, if not impossible. This association between biosecurity and biocontainment is especially pronounced in the aquatic environment, where water, wind, and tidal currents help circulate particulates, wastes, and microorganisms from farm to farm and region to region.

A Maine and New Brunswick based survey of expert opinion (Gustafson et al., 2005) identified the proximity of a farm to a clinical outbreak of ISA as a primary risk factor for subsequent infection with ISAV. Local experts also felt that the time it took to remove an ISAV-infected cage was a predictor of severity of the spread of infection throughout a site. For salmon farms that adhere to biosecurity principles (such as restricting traffic between farms and cleaning, disinfection, and use of site-specific vessels, equipment, gear, and crews), risks associated with geographic proximity to clinical outbreaks may be due to waterborne transfer.

To test this hypothesis previously, water was sampled by USDA APHIS and Micro Technologies, Inc., (Richmond, Maine) from and around a clinical ISAV-positive site from January through June of 2003. ISAV genomic material was repeatedly detected in these water samples, at times over 1 km from the infected site (unpublished data). The persistence (and by extrapolation, infectivity) of ISAV in seawater has been demonstrated in laboratory studies for periods of days to weeks (Nylund et al. 1994; Torgersen 1997; Lovdal and Enger 2002; Giray et al. 2004). Given the substantial mixing from currents and tides in this part of the world (Dowd 2002; Brooks 2003), even 1 day is a theoretically ample time to allow virus particles to travel from an infected site in New Brunswick, Canada to a non-infected site in Maine, or vice versa.

The apparent prevalence of ISAV-infected fish in a cage can increase rapidly over time (Raynard et al. 2001), and even preclinical fish can shed the virus (Totland et al. 1996). A recent field study (Gustafson et al., in press) found a statistically significant relationship between the proportion of RT-PCR positives from subsets of fish sampled during harvest at each of 10 cages (two sites) and mortality rates in the same cages the week prior to harvest. In cages experiencing 0.05% mortality per day, a mortality rate once considered prerequisite to province-officiated depopulation orders (NBDAFA 1998), ISAV was detected in over 10% of sampled harvest fish.

Consequently, removal of infected cages prior to large-scale shedding into a shared water column is presumed to be a critical component to effective disease management of ISA. Field trials and direct empirical studies on the efficacy of early removal, however, are lacking. In this chapter, the authors present results from a retrospective study of nine farm sites designed to evaluate the hypothesis that early removal limits the local spread of ISAV.

Methods

Study site inclusion criteria

Maritime Veterinary Services (MVS) provides veterinary care to a number of salmon farms in both Maine and New Brunswick. Review of all MVS-affiliated sites in Maine and New Brunswick identified nine salmon farms that were diagnosed with ISAV infection during a targeted year class and production cycle. With assurance of confidentiality of site and time identifiers, clients agreed to a review of comprehensive ISAV detection assay records and other factors affecting ISA diagnosis designations. All nine farms that met the inclusion criteria also participated in ISA surveillance activities including veterinary inspections and submission of tissues from moribund fish on a routine basis. During the period of study, barring weather constraints, inspections were conducted at least twice a month (up from once a month) on a farm once ISAV was detected or suspected in any of its cages.

ISAV-infected case definition

Veterinary recommendations for cage removal at times precede a formal diagnosis of ISAV infection based on laboratory tests alone. Consequently, before analyzing the data, the authors established decision criteria to standardize ISAV infection diagnosis dates between farms and cages. A retrospective diagnosis date was defined as the first date that a cage met either of the following two criteria: either (1) two fish were positive by two diagnostic tests or (2) laboratory assays found one fish positive by one test, and were corroborated by any three of the following: (a) a second (different) lab test on any fish from the cage, (b) presumptive clinical signs of ISA in moribund fish, (c) increasing mortality rates (with weekly averages exceeding 0.05% per day), (d) gross pathology consistent with ISA, and/or (e) recent history of ISA on the same or neighboring sites. For example, a farm with prior history of ISA, clinical or gross pathological signs of ISA, and increasing mortality rates (criteria e, b, and c), would only need one confirming laboratory test to meet the definition of an ISAV-positive diagnosis for this study. This system more accurately reflects the actual decision criteria of the practicing veterinarian, and helped to avoid misclassification of cages removed on the basis of veterinary recommendation (rather than delaying for formal laboratory confirmation) that would result from a more stringent definition. Retrospective diagnosis dates were ascribed to dates of sample collection rather than laboratory reporting in all cases.

Data collection

Veterinary and mortality records from each of the nine sites were reviewed to calculate the following: (a) the length of time between ISAV infection diagnosis and harvest (hereafter termed "speed of removal") of the initial (index) positive cage on each site; (b) the time between ISAV infection diagnosis of the index and secondary cages at each site; and (c) the cumulative proportion of surviving (ISAV-negative) cages at each site at 2, 3, and 4 months following diagnosis of the index cage. Calculations of the cumulative proportion of surviving (ISAV-negative) cages were based on Kaplan–Meier estimates of "conditional survival," and account for the number of susceptible cages at risk each interval. To arrive at a cumulative proportion, the number of surviving cages at months-end was first divided by the number of susceptible cages at the beginning of the month for each interval. The proportion surviving month 2 was then multiplied by the proportion surviving month 1 to get cumulative proportion survival for month 2. The proportion surviving month 3 was multiplied by the cumulative survival for month 2 to get cumulative proportion survival for month 3, and so on for month 4.

Data analysis

Statistical associations between the speed of removal and the various severity measures (time between diagnosis of primary and secondary cages, and cumulative proportion of surviving cages at 2, 3, and 4 months following the index diagnosis) were evaluated separately using simple linear regression (Steel et al. 1997). Because of the limited number (4) of follow-up intervals per site, the authors opted for simple linear regression over a time-integrated survival analysis.

Results

The data suggest that speed of removal of the initial infected cage (the "index" cage) on a site can affect the calculated severity measures. Removal time showed a statistically significant association with cumulative percentage of infected cages at 2 months ($p = 0.039$, $R^2 = 47.8$), 3 months ($p = 0.040$, $R^2 = 47.4$), and 4 months ($p = 0.000$, $R^2 = 90.3$) post-diagnosis of the index cage (Figs. 12.1 and 12.2). The tighter association at 4 months results from the loss of one particular farm from the 4-month analysis (due to completion of harvest operations before the 4-month follow-up date). Removal time also showed a loose association ($p < 0.184$, $R^2 = 23.7$) with time to onset of infection in secondary cages (Fig. 12.3).

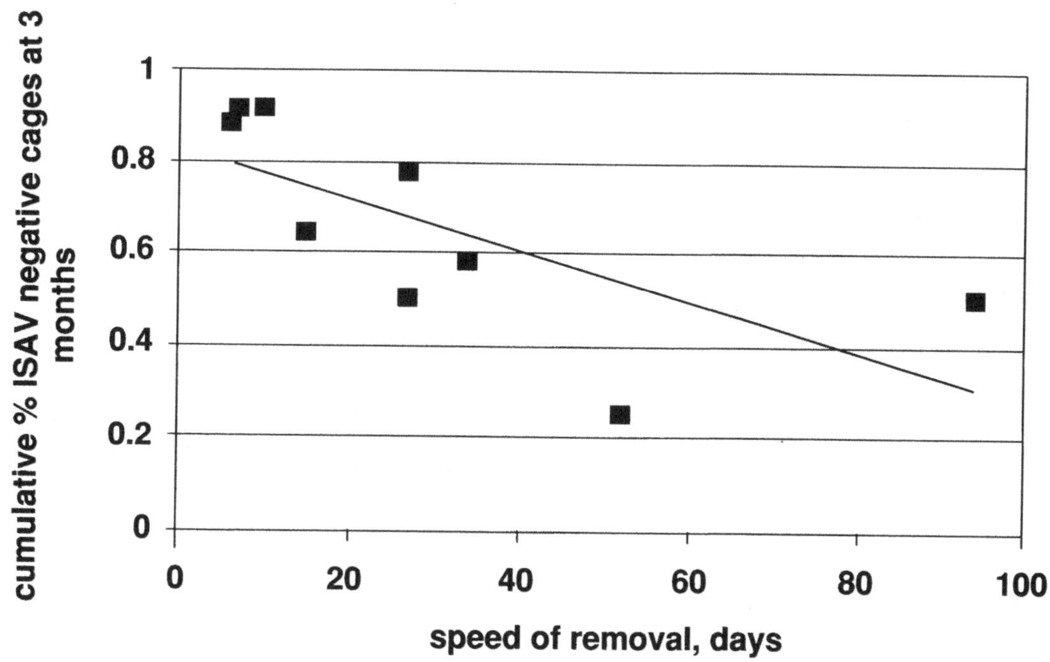

Fig. 12.1 Cumulative 3-month percentage of ISAV-negative cages correlates with speed of removal of the site's index cage. Speed of removal represents the interval between diagnosis and removal of the index cage at a given site. Cumulative % represents the proportion of ISA-negative cages at 3 months post-diagnosis of the index cage. The 2-month post-diagnosis graph looks very similar.

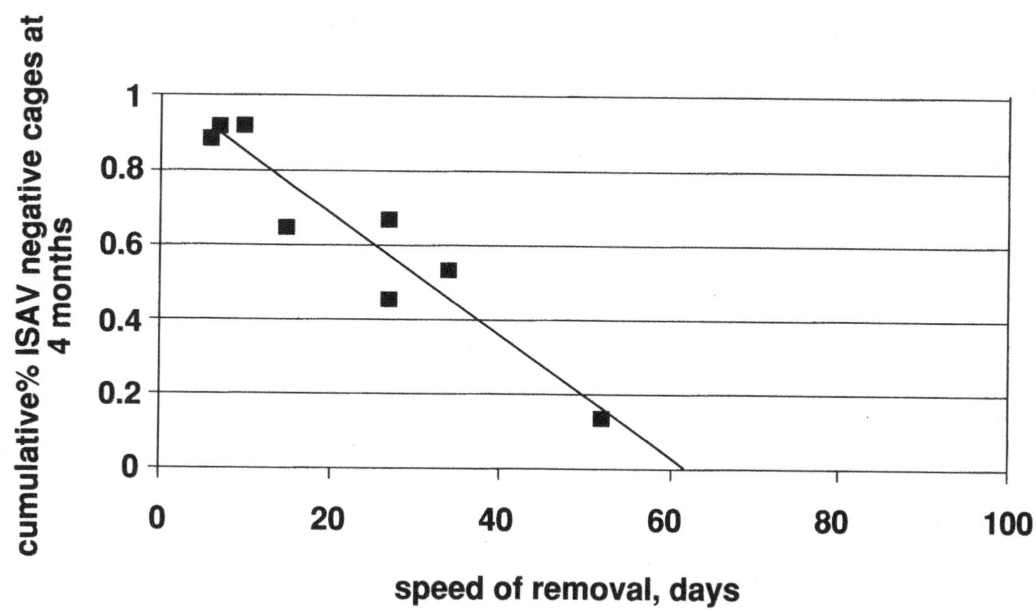

Fig. 12.2 Cumulative 4-month percentage of ISAV-negative cages correlates with the speed of removal of the site's index cage. The *x*-axis represents the interval between diagnosis and removal of the index cage at a given site. The *y*-axis represents the proportion of ISAV-negative cages at 4 months post-diagnosis of the index cage.

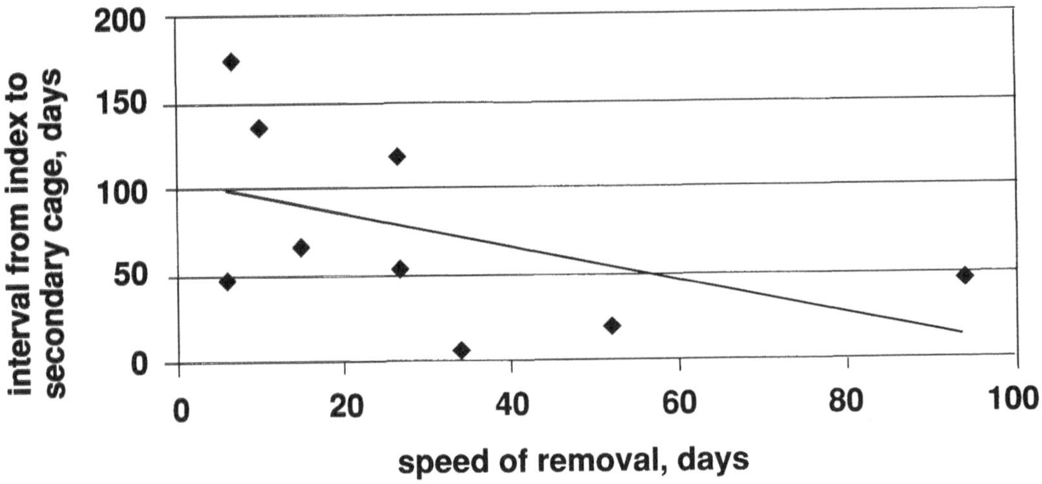

Fig. 12.3 Prompt removal of the index cage may delay the onset of ISA in secondary cages. The *x*-axis represents the interval between diagnosis and removal of the index cage. The *y*-axis represents the length of time between diagnosis of the index and secondary cages.

Conclusions

Early removal of infected cages is considered a key component in the biocontainment of ISA (USDA APHIS Veterinary Services 2002). Early removal, however, is also one of the more difficult control measures for the salmon industry. A typical farm has 8–20 cages on a site, each holding 10–30,000 fish of the same year class. At 4.05 kg (9 lbs) average dressed weight, for example, a market value of U.S.$ 2 per pound would represent an economic return of approximately U.S.$ 500,000 per cage. Loss of even a single cage represents a substantial loss in revenue. In addition, ISAV detection tests vary in sensitivity and specificity (Opitz et al. 2000; McClure et al. 2003; Snow et al. 2003), so early diagnoses are sometimes debated. Furthermore, even recommendations for removal of market-age fish can conflict with market demand, harvest scheduling and vessel availability, drug withdrawal times, or the weather. Though environmental persistence and risk factor studies imply the significance of early removals, the inferred importance of such a dire procedure may not be enough to ensure uniform compliance.

The results of this retrospective study provide initial empirical evidence that early removal is advantageous from a fish health perspective. Sites practicing early removal of ISAV-infected cages showed longer 2-, 3-, and 4-month survival of neighboring cages and possible delays in recurrence of infection. The three sites that removed index cages within 2 weeks of diagnosis showed better survival of remaining cages at 2, 3, and 4 months post-diagnosis than any of the other farms in the study. The authors only evaluated the impact of removal time of the index cage. Removal times of secondary cages were not considered in this preliminary study. Also, the variation in number of cages per site (between 8 and 20) limited resolution of the end-measures of proportional survival, likely reducing statistical power. Despite the limitations in study size and resolution, however, an association between removal time and secondary cages infected was demonstrable.

This work lends initial field support to the theory that prompt removal of infected cages is important to the health and survival of remaining cages on ISAV-infected farms. Further study, however, to test the portability of these conclusions is recommended. Because pathogenicity and host response to viruses, especially Orthomyxoviridae, can vary over time and space, the results demonstrated in this study may not generalize to other settings. The current study is further limited by the exploratory nature of the statistical evaluation, involving independent assessment of a handful of discrete end-points (2, 3, and 4 months post-diagnosis). Future work incorporating more sites and more intervals for follow-up would improve resolution of the end-measures of proportional survival, provide a basis for a fully integrated analysis of survival times, and broaden the applicability of any findings.

Acknowledgments

The authors thank the large number of industry representatives from both Maine and New Brunswick, who have been so helpful with this and other related studies.

References

Bouchard, D.A., K. Brockway, C. Giray, W. Keleher, and P.L. Merrill. 2001. First report of infectious salmon anemia (ISA) in the United States. *Bulletin of the European Association of Fish Pathologists* 21:86–88.

Brooks, D. 2003. *TAMU Coastal Oceanography Modeling Group*. Texas A&M University, Oceanography, College Station, TX. On-line version, http://cobscook.tamu.edu.

Byrne, P.J., D.D. MacPhee, V.E. Ostland, G. Johnson, and H.W. Ferguson. 1998. Haemorrhagic kidney syndrome of Atlantic salmon, *Salmo salar* L. *Journal of Fish Diseases* 21: 81–91.

Dowd, M. 2002. Overview of oceanographic information and approaches: a review of transport and dispersion in coastal waters with reference to the Quoddy region. Pages 36–39 *in* F.H. Page and B.D. Chang, editors. *Fish Health and Oceanography Project of the Aquaculture Collaborative Research and Development Program: Report of the Initial Meeting, 18 December 2001*. Canadian Technical Report of Fisheries and Aquatic Sciences 2409. Fisheries and Oceans Canada, Biological Station, St. Andrews, New Brunswick, Canada.

Giray, C., D.A. Bouchard, K.A. Brockway, and P.L. Merrill. 2004. Environmental persistence of infectious salmon anemia virus. Page 12 *in* S.A. MacLean, editor. *Proceedings of the Second Maine Atlantic Salmon Technical Advisory Committee Research Forum*, 7 January 2004. University of Maine, Orono, ME. National Marine Fisheries Service/Northeast Fisheries Science Center (NMFS/NEFSC), Maine Field Office, Orono, ME.

Gustafson, L.L., S.K. Ellis, and C.A. Bartlett. 2005. Using expert opinion to identify risk factors important to infectious salmon anemia (ISA) outbreaks on salmon farms in Maine, USA and New Brunswick, Canada. *Preventive Veterinary Medicine*. 70(1–2):17–28.

Gustafson, L., S. Ellis, P. Merrill, T. Robinson, and D. MacPhee. In press. Mortality rates predict apparent prevalence of infectious salmon anemia (ISA) at two infected Atlantic salmon farms in Maine. *Bulletin of the European Association of Fish Pathologists*.

Krossoy, B., I. Hordvik, F. Nilsen, A. Nylund, and C. Endresen. 1999. The putative polymerase sequence of infectious salmon anemia virus suggests a new genus within the Orthomyxoviridae. *Journal of Virology* 73:2136–2142.

Lovdal, T. and O. Enger. 2002. Detection of infectious salmon anemia virus in sea water by nested RT-PCR. *Diseases of Aquatic Organisms* 49:123–128.

Lovely, J.E., B.H. Dannevig, K. Falk, L. Hutchin, A.M. MacKinnon, K.J. Melville, E. Rimstad, and S.G. Griffiths. 1999. First identification of infectious salmon anaemia virus in North America with haemorrhagic kidney syndrome. *Diseases of Aquatic Organisms* 35:145–148.

McClure, C.A., K.L. Hammell, I.R. Dohoo, H. Stryhn, and L.J. Hawkins. 2003. Evaluation of infectious salmon anemia diagnostic tests. Pages 69–73 *in* O. Miller and R.C. Cipriano, editors. *International Response in Infectious Salmon Anemia: Prevention, Control, and Eradication.* Proceedings of a Symposium New Orleans, LA, September, 3–4 2002. Technical Bulletin 1902. USDA Animal and Plant Health Inspection Service, Washington, DC. pp. 69–73.

Mjaaland, S., E. Rimstad, K. Falk, and B.H. Dannevig. 1997. Genomic characterization of the virus causing infectious salmon anemia in Atlantic salmon (*Salmo salar* L.): an orthomyxo-like virus in a teleost. *Journal of Virology* 71:7681–7686.

Mullins, J.E., D. Groman, and D. Wadowska. 1998. Infectious salmon anemia in salt water Atlantic salmon (*Salmo salar* L.) in New Brunswick, Canada. *Bulletin of the European Association of Fish Pathologists* 18:110–114.

NBDAFA (New Brunswick Department of Aquaculture, Fisheries and Agriculture). 1998. *Infectious Salmon Anemia (ISAV) Surveillance Program.* St. George, New Brunswick, Canada.

NBDAFA (New Brunswick Department of Aquaculture, Fisheries and Agriculture). 2004. *Infectious Salmon Anemia (ISAV) Surveillance Program.* St. George, New Brunswick, Canada.

Nylund, A., T. Hovland, K. Hodneland, F. Nilsen, and P. Lovik. 1994. Mechanisms for transmission of infectious salmon anaemia (ISA). *Diseases of Aquatic Organisms* 19:95–100.

Opitz, H.M., D. Bouchard, E. Anderson, S. Blake, B. Nicholson, and W. Keleher. 2000. A comparison of methods for the detection of experimentally induced subclinical infectious salmon anaemia in Atlantic salmon. *Bulletin of the European Association of Fish Pathologists* 20:12–22.

Raynard, R.S., M. Snow, and D.W. Bruno. 2001. Experimental infection models and susceptibility of Atlantic salmon *Salmo salar* to a Scottish isolate of infectious salmon anaemia virus. *Diseases of Aquatic Organisms* 47:169–174.

Snow, M., R.S. Raynard, A.G. Murray, D.W. Bruno, J.A. King, R. Grant, I.R. Bricknell, N. Bain, and A. Gregory. 2003. An evaluation of current diagnostic tests for the detection of infectious salmon anaemia virus (ISAV) following experimental water-borne infection of Atlantic salmon, *Salmo salar* L. *Journal of Fish Diseases* 26:135–145.

Steel, R.G.D., J.H. Torrie, and D.A. Dickey. 1997. *Principles and Procedures of Statistics: A Biometrical Approach*, 3rd edition. McGraw-Hill, Boston, MA. 666 pp.

Thorud, K. and H.O. Djupvik. 1988. Infectious anaemia in Atlantic salmon (*Salmo salar* L.) *Bulletin of the European Association of Fish Pathologists* 8:109–111.

Torgersen, Y. 1997. Physical and chemical inactivation of the infectious salmon anemia (ISA) virus. Pages 44–53 *in Proceedings of the Workshop on Infectious Salmon Anaemia.* St. Andrews, New Brunswick, Canada, November 26, 1997. New Brunswick Department of Fisheries and Aquaculture, Fredericton, New Brunswick, Canada.

Totland, G.K., B.K. Hjeltnes, and P.R. Flood. 1996. Transmission of infectious salmon anaemia (ISA) through natural secretions and excretions from infected smolts of Atlantic salmon *Salmo salar* during their presymptomatic phase. *Diseases of Aquatic Organisms* 26:25–31.

USDA APHIS (United States Department of Agriculture, Animal and Plant Health Inspection Service). 2002. *Infectious Salmon Anemia Program Standards.* Final draft, April 30, 2002. United States Department of Agriculture, Animal and Plant Health Inspection Service, Washington, DC. 52 pp.

Index

AAC, 33, 42
OIE Aquatic Animal Health Code, 42
safe trade in aquatic animals, 42
abalone viral mortality, 23, 24
accreditation, 80. *See also* method validation; proficiency testing; reference material production and distribution
competence demonstration by third-party, 81
costs associated with, 83
ILAC, 82
ISO/IEC 17025 requirements for, 82
NACLA system of, 82, 87, 88
reference material, 86
test results and, 82
acid chemical disinfectant, 105
acetic acid ($C_2H_4O_2$), 106
bacteriostatic, 105
carboxylic acids (RCOOH), 106
citric acid ($C_6H_8O_7$), 106
honey, 106
hydrochloric acid, 105
hydrogen ion (H+), 105
mineral acids, 105
sulfuric acid, 105
Acipenser brevirostrum, 41
Acipenser oxyrhynchus, 41
Advisory Group (AG), 24, 26. *See also* aquatic animal health; regional advisory group
Aeromonad hydrophila, 97, 98
Aeromonad septicemia, 97, 98
Aeromonad sobria, 97, 98
Aeromonas salmonicida, 60, 109
Agreement on the Application of Sanitary and Phytosanitary Measures. *See* SPS Agreement
alcoholic antiseptics, 114
alcohols chemical disinfectant, 113–114
aldehydes chemical disinfectant, 111
formaldehyde, 112
glutaraldehyde, 112
Paracide-F, 112
alien aquatic species, 11
alkalis chemical disinfectant (hydroxyl ion), 106
anhydrous sodium carbonate (Na_2CO_3), 106
calcium hydroxide (CaOH), 106
hydrated sodium carbonate ($Na_2CO_3 \cdot 10H_2O$), 106
sodium hydroxide (NaOH), 106
sodium silicate, 106
American Association for Laboratory Accreditation (A2LA), 85, 88
American Association of Veterinary Laboratory Diagnosticians (AAVLD), 87
American Society for Testing and Materials, 84
amphoteric surfactants, 113
Animal and Plant Health Inspection Service, 71
anionic detergents (or non-ionic detergents), 104
anionic surfactants, 113. *See also* surfactants
anthrax spores, 100
antimicrobial spectra, 107, 108
AOAC (Association of Official Analytical Chemists) International, 84
APEC FWG (APEC Fisheries Working Group-funded project), 25
FAO Code of Conduct for Responsible Fisheries, 25
FAO Regional Technical Cooperation Programme, 25
FAO/NACA Regional project, 25
NACA/FAO/OIE Asia-Pacific QAAD reporting system, 25
WTO's Sanitary and Phytosanitary Agreement, 25
WWF/FAO/NACA Consortium on Shrimp and the Environment, 25
Aphanomyces invadans/piscicida, 19
approvals, 80. *See also* competence
aquaculture. *See also* biosecurity
abalone mortalities, 18
as food producing sector, 11, 17
disease threats, 9
diseases and pathogens, 18
FAO statistics, 11
health maintenance, 10
in Asia-Pacific region, 18
role of alien aquatic species and genotypes, 11
shrimp aquaculture (small-scale), 14
aquatic animal disease, diagnosis of, 77–88. *See also* accreditation; aquatic animal biosecurity; competence; laboratory systems; method validation

aquatic animal disease, diagnosis of *(Continued)*
eradication of, 3
prevention and control of, 3–8
Aquatic Code, 5
OIE, 3
reporting system (QAAD), 22
spread of
abalone mortalities, 18
carp mortalities, 18
economic losses, 18
KHV losses, 18
aquatic animal health
activities (Canada), 37
Asia regional advisory group, 26
disease outbreak in Asia, 18
EUS, 18
regional resource base, 26
surveillance for, 129–43
trans-boundary movement, 18
Aquatic Animal Health Code, 4, 12
Aquatic Animal Health Diagnostic Systems, 77
aquatic animal health information management system, 139
Canada's fishery (general) regulations, 37
FAO, 17
fish health protection regulations, 36
health management protocols, 18
individual client information, 139
international disease reporting, 139
Malpeque disease, 33–36
national disease reporting system, 139
national network, 139
OIE, 17
pathogens, 10
regional approach, 17
salmonid aquaculture, 36–37
Aquatic Animal Health Office, 37, 40
Aquatic Animal Health Policy (AAHP), 55–67
aquatic animal health program (Canada), 40, 41, 42, 155–162. *See also* infectious hematopoietic necrosis
Aquatic Animal Health Research Institute (AAHRI), 18
Aquatic Animal Health Standards Commission, 4, 33
aquatic animal health surveillance, 129–143
certification of exports, 129
components of, 134, 136–139
design and structure of, 134
diseases detection, 129
effective aquatic animal emergency disease preparedness, 130
endemic diseases control, 129, 130
flow-through conditions, 130
general surveillance, 132
implementation of, 141
international reporting, 129
list of diseases of concern, 136
mechanism of, 134
objectives of, 131, 134–136
requirements of, 133
risk analysis, 129
sound aquatic animal health advice to farmers, 129
spread of aquatic animal pathogens risk reduction, 129, 130
surveillance components, 132
targeted surveillance, 132, 133
types of
active, 132
general, 132
passive, 132
scanning, 132
targeted, 132
aquatic animal pathogen spread, 17
Aquatic Animals Commission, 4
Aquatic Code, 3, 4, 5, 6, 7, 12, 13, 42, 140
Aquatic Manual, 5
aquatic species health maintenance, 91
biosecurity, 91
disinfection, 91
Aquatic Veterinary Medicine Committee, 70
Asia regional advisory group on aquatic animal health, 26
Asia Regional Technical Guidelines, 17, 21, 22, 26
and Beijing Consensus and Implementation Strategy, 21
and CCRF, 21
and companion documents, 21
and FAO, 21
and NACA, 21
and OIE, 21
and TCP/RAS 6714 and 9605, 21
and WTOSPS Agreement, 21
Asia Diagnostic Guide to Aquatic Animal Diseases, 21
contingency planning, 21
disease diagnosis, 21
disease surveillance and reporting, 21
disease zoning, 21
guiding principles, 21
health certification, 21
implementation of, 21, 22
IRA, 21
managing risk associated with
live aquatic animals movement, 21
trans-boundary pathogens, 21
Manual of Procedures, 21
national strategies, 21
on health management, 21
pathogens, 21
policy frameworks, 21
quarantine measures, 21
regional capacity building, 21
Technical Guidelines regional AG on aquatic animal health, 26

Asia-Pacific Economic Cooperation (APEC), 18
Asia-Pacific quarterly aquatic animal disease reporting (NACA/FAO/OIE list), 22–24
mass mortalities, 24
NACA/FAO/OIE disease list, 22
NACA/FAO/OIE QAAD-Asia-Pacific reporting system, 22
NACA/OIE Expert Consultation recommendation, 22
non-OIE-listed, 23
OIE-listed, 23
QAAD, 22, 24
unknown diseases of serious nature, 23
Association of Official Analytical Chemists, 94
effectiveness tests, 94
HBV, 94
HCV, 94
herpes, 94
HIV, 94
Association of Southeast Asian Nations (ASAN), 18
Atlantic haddock, 41
Atlantic halibut, 41
Atlantic salmon, 155. *See also* Pacific salmon
Atlantic salmon farms (Maine), 165
infectious hematopoietic necrosis (IHN), 155–62
lack of biosecurity awareness consequences, example of, 150
Atlantic sturgeon, 41
Aulorhynchus flavidus, IHN in, 157
Australian Agency for International Aid (AusAID), 18
Australian Centre for International Agricultural Research (ACIAR), 18
autoclaveing, 101
awareness, biosecurity. *See* biosecurity awareness

Bacillus anthrasis, 105
bacterial gill disease (*F. branchiophila*), 97, 98
bacterial kidney disease (BKD), 96, 98
bay scallops, 41
Beijing Consensus and Implementation Strategy, 21
beta radiation physical disinfectant, 102
better management practices (BMPs), 14. *See also* good management practices
beverage pasteurization, 101
biguanides, 106–107
biosecurity, 9–12
and agriculture, 10–12
animal pests, 10
aquatic animal disease diagnosis aspects, 77–88
aquatic animal pathogens, 17
as risk with food and agriculture, 10
at farm level, 15
awareness, 150–154
BMP, 15
diseases, 10
farm level, 149–162
genotypes management, 10
GMO, 10
harmonization of standards and procedures, 12
in agriculture, 10
in developing countries, 13–14
in Food and agriculture markets, 12
infectious hematopoietic necrosis (IHN), 155–162
international measures, 13
invasive alien species management, 10
ISA, 166
opportunities and challenges for developing countries, 9
plant pests, 10
protocol development, 12
risk management, 10
risk-assessment worksheets (U.S.), 56–67
shrimp disease control, 14
international instruments, 9
international measures, 12
zoonoses, 10
blood-borne pathogens, 95
blue and gallo mussels, 38
Bonamia exitiosus, 20
brain parasite, 72
British Columbia Fish Health Policy (FHPR requirements), 38
British Columbia MAFF (BCMAFF), 38, 155, 161. *See also* infectious hematopoietic necrosis
and DFO, 38
wild fish health research, 161
Brucella abortus, 101

calibration laboratories, 82. *See also* laboratory systems
Canada
aquatic animal biosecurity, 31–54, 155–162
aquatic animal health activities, 37–40
aquatic animal health management, 33–37
aquatic animal health program, 40, 41, 42, 155–162
international change, 41
national changes, 40
aquatic biosecurity, 31–32
aquatic environment disease prevention, 32–33
Canada's Fishery Act (FHPR), 37
endangered marine mammal populations, 39
federal system, 37
fish health protection regulations (FHPR), 36, 37
Fisheries Act, 37
ICES Code of Practice, 41
MSX (case study), 43
national aquatic animal health partnership (NAAHP), 42, 43
scallop production, 41
zonation, 49
Canada's Fishery Act (FHPR), 37

Canadian Council of Fisheries and Aquaculture Ministers (CCFAM), 42
Cape Breton oysters, 36
carcasses composting, 101
cartagena protocol, 13
cationic bisbiguanide, 106
cationic detergents (or invert soaps), 104
cationic surfactants, 112, 113
Catostomus commersoni, 75
caustic soda, 106
CBD (Convention on Biological Diversity), 13
CDC (Centers for Disease Control), 93, 94
  and EPA, 94
    with tuberculocidal claim, 94
    without tuberculocidal claim, 94
  and FDA, 94
ceratomyxosis (CS) parasite, 96, 98
CFIA (Canadian Food Inspection Agency), 39
Chemical Abstract Service (CAS), 103
chemical disinfectant, 95, 100, 103–114
  acids, 105
  alcohols, 113
  aldehydes, 111
  alkalis, 106
  biguanides, 106
  CAS, 103
  chemical registry, 103
  detergent, 103
  dyes, 114
  gas, 114
  halogens, 107
  heavy metals, 114
  oxidizing agents, 110
  peracetic acid, 110
  phenols, 104
  soaps/detergents, 103
  surfactants, 112
  Virkon S®, 111
chemical registry, 103
Chloramine T, sporicidal action, 108
chlorhexidine, 107
chlorinated lime, 108
CITAC 1998, 83
Code of Conduct for Responsible Fisheries (CCRF), 21
Code of Federal Regulations (CFR), 93
Codex Alimentarius Commission, 13
coldwater disease (*Flexibacter psychrophilus*), 97, 98
Columnaris (*Flexibacter columnaris*), 97, 98
Commonwealth Scientific and Industrial Research Organization (CSIRO), 18
competence
  demonstration, 80
    by third-party accreditation, 81
  recognition, 80, 86
  verification, 80
composting, 101
convention on biological diversity, 13
Cooperation on International Traceability in Analytical Chemistry, 84
Crassostrea gigas, 32, 37, 38, 41
Crassostrea virginica, 32, 33, 35, 41, 47, 133
Creutzfeldt-Jakob disease agents, 94
Cymatogaster aggregata, 157. *See also* IHN
Cyprinus carpio, 18

demand-release chlorine dioxide
  in chlorination, 107
Denman Island Disease, 37
detergent chemical disinfectant, 103
  anionic, 104
  cationic, 104
DFO, 37, 40
  AAH, 40
  and BCMAFF, 38
  as competent authority, 40
  CCFAM, 42
  FHPR, 40
  FWI, 37
  GFC, 37
  marine mammal pathology, 39
  NRAAH, 40
  PBS, 37
diagnostic data and test result validity. *See* accreditation; laboratory systems
digenean flukes, 72
disease emergencies, 26, 27
diseases and pathogens, 18
  biosecurity, 3–8, 9–16, 91
  blood-borne, 95
  EUS, 18
  finfish diseases, 19
  KHV, 18
  molluscan diseases, 20
  shrimp diseases, 20
  TSV, 18
  VER, 18
  WSSV, 18
disinfectants. *See also* chemical disinfectant; physical disinfectant
  against pathogens, 91
  antiseptic, 91
  application of, 115, 118
  CDC, 94
  discharge of, 92
  disposal, 92, 119
  efficacy and characteristics of, 92
  germicide, 91, 92, 95
  impact, 103
  steam as, 100
  US regulatory framework, 93
    EPA, 93
    FDA, 93

disinfection protocols (MDIF&W), 119–21
  cleanliness, 121
  dead fish disposal procedure, 119
  equipment disinfection procedure, 119
  footbaths, 120–21
  for IHN, 157
  hatchery tools, 121
  hatchery visitors, 121
  spray disinfection procedure, 119
  stocking trucks, well boats, tenders, and feed barges, 121
disposal policy, disinfectant, 92
DNR (Department of Natural Resources), 69
downtime, 118
dry heat disinfection, 101
dyes chemical disinfectant, 114

eggs and gametes movement, 13
Emergency Disease Control Task Force, 27
emulsifier, 103
endemic diseases, 136
enteric redmouth (*Yersinia ruckerii*) BR, 96, 98
enveloped viruses, 100, 105, 112
EPA (Environmental Protection Agency), 92
  AOAC effectiveness tests, 94
  disinfectant, 93
    classification, 94
    products list, 95
    registration, 94
epitheliocystis, 24
epizootic ulcerative syndrome, 18, 19
equipment disinfection procedure, 119
Escherichia coli, 101
Esox lucius, 112
European Inland Fisheries Advisory Commission (EIFAC), 13, 140
EUS (epizootic ulcerative syndrome), 19
exotic diseases (OIE-listed), 136
  finfish diseases, 23
  mollusc diseases, 23

fallowing, 5
FAO (Food and Agricultural Organization), 15, 18, 32
  FAO/NACA/OIE regional QAAD reporting list
  molluscan health management, 24
  trans-boundary movement, 32
farm level biosecurity, 149–62
  awareness, 152–54
    importance of, 150–52
    in farm staff, 149
  farm staff and
    communication channels, maintaining of, 154
    fish health-related aspects, 153
    motivational and sense of pride related aspects, 153
    standard operating procedures (SOPs) and systems for, 153
    training of, 153
    up-to-date industry knowledge, 154
farmed Atlantic salmon, IHN in, 155–162
FDA
  and CDC guidelines, 94
  disinfectants, 93
    classification, 94
    in health-care settings, 93
Federal Insecticide, Fungicide, and Rodenticide Act (FIFRA), 93
federal system (Canada), 37
FHPR (Fish Health Protection Regulations), 37
FHPR Manual of Compliance, 40
finfish diseases, 19–20
fish health centers (FHCs), 56
fish health maintenance program, 122
Fish Health Management Plan, 160
Fish Health Officials (FHOs), 39
Fish Health Plans, 155
Fish Health Policy, 56
fish health problems, 75
fish health protection regulations (Canada), 36, 37
Fish Health Section of the American Fisheries Society (AFS-FHS), 81
fish health standards (WDATCP), 75
Fish Health Unit, 39
Fish Health, Veterinary Approach, 69–76
fish pathogens, 92
  Aeromonad septicemia (*Aeromonad hydrophila*, *Aeromonad sobria*), 98
  bacterial gill disease (*F. branchiophila*), 98
  bacterial kidney disease (BKD), 98
  ceratomyxosis (CS) parasite, 98
  classification, 96
Fisheries Act, 37
Fishery (General) Regulation of Canada, 37
flexibacter, 72
Food and Agricultural Organization (FAO), 11, 17, 149
Food and Drug Administration, 84, 92
food safety, 13
footbaths, 120–21
formaldehyde, 112
FTCs (fish technology centers), 56
Furunclulosis (*Aeromonas salmonicida*) BF, 96, 98
FWI (Freshwater Institute), 38, 39
FWI Fish Health Unit, 38
FWR, 37, 38
  CCWHC, 38
  fish kill investigation, 38
  fish products certification, 38
  FWI, 38
FWS Form, 57, 60

Gadus morhua, 41
gamma radiation physical disinfectant, 102

gas chemical disinfectants, 114
beta-propiolactone, 115
ethylene oxide (C_2H_4O), 114
formaldehyde, 115
methylbromide (CH_3Br), 115
ozone (O_3), 115
propylene oxide (C_3H_6O), 115
geoduck abscess lesions, 38
geographic information systems, 137
germicide, 91, 92, 95
GFC (Gulf Fisheries Centre), 39
GIS (geographic information systems), 137–139
GMO (genetically modified organisms), 10
good management practices (GMPs), 36. *See also* better management practices
GPS (geographic positioning system), 40
Gram-negative bacteria, 107, 113
Gram-positive bacteria, 94, 107
Great Lakes Fish Health Committee, 38
grouper iridoviral disease, 20, 24
Gulf Fisheries Centre, 37
Gyrodactylus, 72

haemic neoplasias, 38
Haliotis diversicolor, 20
Haliotis kamtschatkana, 41
halogens chemical disinfectant, 107
calcium hypochlorite ($Ca(OCl)_2$), 108, 109
Chloramine T, 107, 108
demand-release chlorine dioxide, 107
effect of pH, 107
exposure to fish, 108
hypochlorite, 107, 108
hypochlorous acid, 107
iodine, 109, 110
iodophors, 109
organic matter presence, 107
sodium dichloroisocyanurate, 107, 108
sodium hypochlorite, 107
sodium thiosulfate, 107
with ammonia, 108
with phosphoric acid, 108
Haplosporidium nelsoni, 20, 23, 31, 34, 44, 50, 133
Haplosporidium costale, 47, 50
hatchery, 121
health management (Asia Regional Technical Guidelines), 21
heat physical disinfectant, 95–101
biomedical waste incineration, 101
carcass incineration, 101
composting, 101
dry heat, 101
flaming bacterial inoculation loops, 101
ISA, 100
moist heat, 100, 101
protein coagulation, 100
searing, 101
steam cleaning, 100
heavy metals chemical infectants, 114
copper salts, 114
organic mercury, 114
silver nitrate, 114
zinc salts, 114
hemic neoplasia, 39
hemorrhaging fish example, biosecurity awareness and, 151
herpes, 94
heterosporis, 72
high efficiency particulate air (HEPA), 103
Hippoglossus hippoglossus, 41
hospital disinfectants, 94
HTH, 119
human immunodeficiency virus (HIV), 94
hydrographic circulation, 34. *See also* Malpeque Bay disease
hypochlorite, 108, 119

ICES (International Council for the Exploration of the Sea), 13, 36, 140
Ichthyophonus hoferi outbreak, 36
Ictalurus punctatus, 112
IHN (infectious haematopoietic necrosis), 38, 155–162
2001 outbreak, 156–157
disinfection protocol for, 157
future scope, 158–162
short-term outcomes, 159
IHNV, 157
in Atlantic salmon (*Salmo salar* L.), 155, 156
in Pacific salmon (*Oncorhynchus* spp.), 155, 156
regulatory role in, 160
research scope in, 160
risk factors, 157–158
vaccine for, 158
wild fish health research, 161
IHNV (infectious hematopoietic necrosis virus), 96, 98, 156, 157, 159, 161
impact physical disinfectant (explosives), 103
import risk analysis (IRA), 5, 25
indirect fluorescent antibody technique (IFAT), 166
infected cages removal, 165–172. *See also* ISA
infectious hematopoietic necrosis (IHN), 3–8, 155–162
infectious salmon anemia, 31, 50, 100, 166
International Code on Aquatic Animal Health, 37
International Cooperation for Laboratory Accreditation (ILAC), 80, 81
guidelines for reference material production and distribution, 86
ILAC 2000a standard, 86
ILAC 2000b standard, 85
laboratories accreditation and, 82

International Council for the Exploration of the Sea, 13, 36
international disease reporting, 139, 140
International Electrotechnical Commission (IEC), 81
International Plant Protection Convention (IPPC), 13
International Union of Pure and Applied Chemistry, 84
invasive alien species, CBD, 13
iodophor
  povidone-iodine, 109
  radiation as disinfectants, 102
IPNV (infectious pancreatic necrosis virus), 96, 98
iridoviral disease, 24
ISA (infectious salmon anemia), 50, 100
  biocontainment, 166, 170
  biosecurity, 166
  cell culture, 166
  data analysis, 168
  early removal of infected cages, 170
  IFAT, 166
  infected cage removal, 165
  ISAV, 166–170
  Maine and New Brunswick based survey, 166
  market-age fish removal, 170
  MVS, 167
  orthomyxoviridae, 166
  RT-PCR, 166
  salmon farms, 166
  single cage loss, 170
  veterinary and mortality records, 168
ISA virus (ISAV), 96, 98, 165–168
ISO, 80
ISO 1997a, 1997b standards, 85. *See also* proficiency testing
ISO 2000a standard, 83, 86
ISO 9000 standards (ISO 2000b, 2000c, 2000d), 82
ISO Guide 34, 86
ISO/IEC 17025 standard, 82, 83, 84, 87, 88. *See also* accreditation
ITCs (Introductions and Transfers Committees), 39

Japanese scallops, 38

koi herpes virus, 18–20, 24
Kudoa, 38

laboratory systems, 78–80
  AAVLD, 87
  accreditation systems
    ILAC, 82
    international and national, 80
    NACLA, 82, 87
  approvals, 80
  competence areas, 79, 80, 81
  ISO/IEC 17025 requirements, 86
largemouth bass, 72
Lepomis macrochirus, 112
LFHO (Local Fish Health Officers), 39
lipophilic viruses, 107
Litopenaeus vannamei, 20
live brood stock, 12
LMOs (living genetically modified organisms), 13

Macrobrachium rosenbergii, 20
Maine Department of Inland Fisheries and Wildlife, 101
malachite green, 114
Malpeque Bay disease, 31, 33–36
Manual of Diagnostic Tests for Aquatic Animals, 4, 140
Marine Products Export Development Authority (MPEDA), 14
Marteilia sydneyi, 20, 23
Marteilioides chungmuensis, 23, 24
mass mortalities, 20
  common carp, 18, 24
  Crassostrea virginica, 33
  koi, 18, 20, 23, 24
  Malpeque disease, 33
  of *Clupea harengus harengus*, 36
  small abalone, 20
  soft-shell clams (*Mya arenaria*), 39
Material Safety Data Sheet, 111
MDIF, 119–121
Mekong River Commission (MRC), 18
Melanogrammus aeglefinus, 41
Mercenaria mercenaria, 41
method validation. *See also* accreditation
  defined, 83
  ISO 2004a, 83
  ISO/IEC 17025, 83, 84
Micropterus salmoides, 72, 112
microwave radiation physical disinfectant, 102
Mikrocytos mackini suppression, 38
moist heat disinfection, 102
molluscan diseases, 20, 24
Mourilyan virus, 20
MSDS (Material Safety Data Sheet), 111
MSX, 34, 39
  infection, 47
  positive zone, 48
  zonation, 49
mullet iridoviral disease, 24
muscle parasite, 72
MVS (Maritime Veterinary Services), 167
Mya arenaria, 39, 41
Mycobacterium bovis, 101
Mycobacterium tuberculosis, 95
mycotic granulomatosis, 19. *See* EUS
Mytilus edulis, 38, 41, 46
Mytlius galloprovincialis, 38
Myxobolus neurophilus, 72

NAAHP (national aquatic animal health program), 42, 43
NACA (Network of Aquaculture Centres in Asia-Pacific), 14, 17, 18
AAHRI, 18
ACIAR, 18
and FAO Aquatic Animal Pathogen and Quarantine information system, 25
APEC, 18, 25
aquatic animal health, 17, 21
ASEAN, 18
Asia regional advisory group on aquatic animal health, 26
Asia Regional Technical Guidelines, 17, 21
Asia-Pacific quarterly aquatic animal disease reporting system, 22–24
AusAID, 18
CSIRO, 18
disease control, 21
disease emergency, 26
implementation of Technical Guidelines, 22
import risk analysis (IRA), 25
information and capacity building, 24
molluscan health management, 24
MRC, 18
regional programs and outputs, 20
regional resource base for aquatic animal health, 26
response to disease emergencies, 26
rural development, 21
SEAFDEC, 18
sustainable aquaculture, 21
NACA/FAO/OIE, 19, 22, 23, 24
NACA/OIE/FAO list, 141
NACA's Third Five-Year Work Programme (2001–2005), 21
National Animal Health Emergency Monitoring System, 86
National Animal Health Laboratory Network (NAHLN) laboratories, 79, 86
National Committee for Clinical Laboratory Standards, 84
National Cooperation for Laboratory Accreditation (NACLA), 80, 81, 82, 88
national disease reporting system, 139
National Registry of Aquatic Animal Health, 40
National Registry of Fish Diseases, 40
National Strategy on Aquatic Animal Health, 22
National Technology Transfer and Advancement Act (NTTAA) of 1996, 80
Network of Aquaculture Centres in Asia-Pacific, 14, 17
NFHS (National Fish Hatchery System), 56
nocardiosis, 38
non-enveloped viruses, 105, 106, 112
non-ionic surfactants, 113
non-OIE-listed diseases, 23
non-pathognomic, 32
non-routine testing, 83
non-salmonid fish health assessment, 72
Northumberland Strait, 34. *See also* Malpeque Bay disease
nosocomial pathogen, 94
Notemigonus crysoleucas, 75
NRAAH (National Registry of Aquatic Animal Health)
as coordination center, 40
database, web-based, 40
DFO Science web-site, 40
FHPR health reports, 40
FHPR Manual of Compliance revision, 40
salmonid health certification, 40

Occupational Safety and Health Administration, 93
OES (occupational exposure limit), 111
OIE (Office International des Èpizooties), 3–7, 12, 13, 17–26, 32, 33, 37, 39, 40, 42–46, 48, 78, 79, 81, 82, 84, 130, 131, 133, 135, 136, 139, 140, 141
AAC, 33, 42
and KHV and grouper iridoviral disease, 20
disease reporting, 140
diseases listed in, 12
guidelines for aquatic animal surveillance, 140
international disease reporting, 140
normative works, 3
objectives of, 4
PBS, 37
standards of, 4–5
world trade safeguard, 3
OIE Aquatic Animal Health Code, 12, 22, 42
health standards, 12
genetic material diseases, 12
live aquatic animals movement, 12
OIE Aquatic Animal Health Standards, 21
OIE Aquatic Code, 37, 40, 42
OIE International Committee, 4
OIE Terrestrial Animal Health Standards Commission, 4
OIE-listed diseases, 23
Oncorhychus mykiss, 109
Oncorhynchus masou virus (OMV), 96, 98
Oncorhynchus mykiss, 40, 60
Oncorhynchus nerka, 157
Oncorhynchus spp., 36, 40
IHN in, 155, 156
OSHA (Occupational Safety and Health Administration), 93
EPA, 94
occupational exposure to blood-borne pathogens, 94
workplace standards, 93
Ostrea conchaphila, 37

Ostrea edulis, 32, 38, 41
oxidizing agents chemical disinfectant, 110

Pacific salmon, 155, 156. *See also* Atlantic salmon; infectious hematopoietic necrosis
Panope abrupta, 41
passive surveillance, 132
pasteurization, 100. *See also* beverage pasteurization
Patinopecten yessoensis, 38, 41
PBS (Pacific Biological Station), 37, 38, 39
PBS Fish Health Unit, 38
PEI (Prince Edward Island), 33
Penaeus monodon, 20
peracetic acid chemical disinfectant, 110, 111
Perca flavescens, 70
Perkinsus marinus, 49
Perkinsus olseni, 20, 23
Perkinsus qugwadi, 38
phenols chemical disinfectant, 104
  bleach dilution, 104
  carbolic acid, 105
  cresylic acid, 105
  effect of temperature, 105
  hyperbilirubinemia, 105
  in concentrated solutions, 105
  ineffective against, 105
  lipophilic viruses, 104
  residual films, 104
  skin depigmentation, 104
  substituted phenol, 105
phylogenetic affinities, 38
physical disinfectant
  as sunlight, 101
  beta and gamma radiation, 102
  filtration, 102, 103
  heat as, 95–101
  impact, 103
  microwave radiation, 102
  ultraviolet light, 102
Pimephales promelas, 75
Placopecten magellanicus, 41
Pleuronectes americanus, 41
post-stocking management, 15
proficiency testing, 84. *See also* accreditation; method validation; reference material production and distribution
proliferative kidney disease (PKX), 96, 98
Prosorhynchus squamatous, 39
protistan parasite, 31
Protothaca staminea, 41
pseudo kidney disease (*Lactobacillus* sp.), 97, 98
Pseudomonas aeruginosa, 94
put-and-take rainbow trout, 40

QAAD (Quarterly Aquatic Animal Disease), 19, 22, 24
quarantine, 21, 41
quaternary ammonium compounds (quats), 112, 113, 119

red spot disease. *See* EUS
reference material production and distribution, 85, 86. *See also* accreditation; method validation; proficiency testing
regional advisory group, 26
Regional Aquatic Animal Health Resource Base, 26
regional disease reporting system. *See* Asia-Pacific quarterly aquatic animal disease reporting system
regional reference laboratories (RRL), 26
regional resource experts (RRE), 26
Regional Technical Guidelines (Asia), 21
resistance mechanisms, 115
rickettsial-like agent, 41
risk classification, 60
risk-assessment worksheets, 57–60, 64
rotovirus, 104
Royal Society of Canada by Needler and Logie (1947), 33
RRC (regional resource centres), 26

Salmo salar, 31, 36, 40, 100, 109
  IHN in, 155, 156
  lack of biosecurity awareness consequences, example of, 150
Salmo trutta, 109
salmon anemia, spread of infectious, 165–72
salmon farms, 166
Salmonella choleraesuis, 94
salmonid aquaculture, 36–37, 92, 166
Salvelinus aureus, 110
Salvelinus fontinalis, 109
Salvelinus namaycush, 109
sanitary and phytosanitary measures agreement, 13
scallop production (Canada), 41
SCUBA, 32
sea-side organism (SSO), 32
Serratia marcescens, 113
shellfinfish diagnostics, 39
Shellfish Health Unit, 39
shortnose sturgeon, 41
shrimp aquaculture, small-scale, 14
shrimp disease, 20
  epidemiological approach, 14
  MPEDA, 14
  NACA, 14
small abalone, 20
soaps chemical disinfectant, 103
soda ash, 106
sodium dichloroisocyanurate, 108
sodium lauryl sulfate (SLS), 104
Southeast Asian Fisheries Development Center (SEAFDEC), 18
SPG, 38

spherical baculovirosis (*Penaeus monodon*-type baculovirus), 23
sporicidal disinfectant, 105, 106
spotted prawn disease, 38
spray disinfection procedure, 119
spring viremia of carp, 72
SPS Agreement, 3, 4, 13, 25, 33, 41, 42
  and WTO, 13
standard operating procedures (SOPs), farm-level biosecurity and, 153
steam disinfection, 100
sterilants, 93
Stizostedion vitreum, 75
Streptococcus infection (*Streptococcus innaea*), 97, 98
Strongylocentrotus droebachiensis, 41
sunlight physical disinfectant, 101
surface disinfection, 110
surfactants
  anionic surfactants, 113
  as chemical disinfectant, 112, 113
  cationic surfactants, 113
  sodium lauryl sulfate (SLS), 104
surgical antiseptic, 105
surveillance. *See* aquatic animal health surveillance
sustainable aquaculture, 21

Tapes philippinarum, 41
targeted surveillance, 132, 133
Taura syndrome virus (TSV), 18, 20
TBQR, 119
Technical Guidelines. *See* Asia Regional Technical Guidelines
testing. *See* proficiency testing
topical antiseptics, 114
trans-boundary aquatic animal, 13, 21
  and APEC, 25
  Asia Regional Technical Guidelines, 21
  Beijing Consensus and Implementation Strategy, 21
  carp mass mortalities, 18
  cartagena protocol, 13
  disease outbreak in Asia, 18
  KHV, 18
  koi mass mortalities, 18
  NACA/ FAO/OIE, 19
Trichodina, 72
tuberculocidal claim, 95

U.S. Fish & Wildlife Service, 55–67
ulcerative mycosis. *See* EUS
ultraviolet light physical disinfectant, 102
U.S. Department of Agriculture, Animal and Plant Health Inspection Service (USDA-APHIS), 81, 87
USFWS Form, 58

vaccine, IHN, 158
validation, defined, 83. *See also* accreditation; laboratory systems; method validation
Variola major, 94
Veterinary Approach (Wisconsin), fish health, 69–76
veterinary certification, 71
veterinary disinfectants, 114
Vibriosis (*Vibrio anguillarum*, *Vibrio salmonicida*), 97, 98
VIMS (Virginia Institute of Marine Sciences), 44, 45
viral encephalopathy and retinopathy (VER), 18, 19
Viral hemorrhagic septicemia virus (VHSV), 96, 98
Virkon S® chemical disinfectant, 111

WDATCP, 69
  aquaculture veterinarians, 72
  certification of veterinarians, 69
  communication among stakeholders, 76
  fish farms registration, 71
  fish health program, 70
  fish import permits, 75
  harmonization of fish health regulations, 76
  health standards rules, 69
  non-salmonid fish health assessment, 72
  registration of fish farms, 69
  science-based best management standards, 76
  success of, 75
  veterinarians certification, 71, 72
WDATCP Fish Health Program, 70
web-based NRAAH database, 40
wet washing, 116
whirling disease (*Myxobolus cerebralis*) (WD), 97, 98
white spot disease (WSD), 14, 18, 20, 23
winter flounder, 41
Wisconsin (USA) Department of Agriculture, Trade and Consumer Protection (WDATCP), 69
Wisconsin Veterinary Approach, fish health, 69–76
Wisconsin yellow perch, 72
World Organisation for Animal Health, 32, 78
World Wildlife Fund (WWF), 25
WSSV (white spot syndrome virus), 18, 20
WTO (World Trade Organization), 4, 13, 130
  SPA Agreement (Sanitary and Phytosanitary Agreement), 4, 21, 25, 33

yellow head disease, 23
yellow perch, 70, 72, 75
Yersinia pestis, 94
Yersinia ruckeri, 109

zonation, 40, 49, 130
zoonoses, 4, 10, 39

Printed and bound by CPI Group (UK) Ltd, Croydon, CR0 4YY
16/09/2026
14963448-0004